THE BABY BOOK

'There is no family, no father or mother who does not experience worry. Anyone who denies this is either deliberately not telling the truth, or cannot recognise the truth. Our success depends to a large extent on our attitudes to the problems which all of us face and less to the problems themselves. There is no getting away from the fact that it is hard work. There is no denying that to achieve a good family compromise, some of our own individual activities must for a while take second place.

'The family who denies that the coming of children makes a difference, that they must not be allowed to rule your life, is wrong. They do make a difference; particularly on mobility and holidays, and the ease of taking either your own special hobby or the shared evenings and outings with your spouse. If you used to enjoy a weekly trip to the cinema, you should continue this after the first week or two and when you have made adequate baby-sitting arrangements. Being a family person is certainly a more selfless existence than being alone. But the rewards are numerous.'

Extract from the author's Introduction

THE
BABY BOOK

Rosemary Sturgess

MAGNUM BOOKS
Methuen Paperbacks Ltd

A Magnum Book

THE BABY BOOK
ISBN 0 417 03160 2

First published in Great Britain 1977
by David & Charles Limited
Magnum edition published 1979

copyright © 1977 by Rosemary Sturgess

Magnum Books are published
by Methuen Paperbacks Ltd
11 New Fetter Lane, London EC4P 4EE

Made and printed in Great Britain
by Richard Clay (The Chaucer Press) Ltd
Bungay, Suffolk

To John with thanks

THE BABY BOOK

CONTENTS

INTRODUCTION

There are few more absorbing pastimes than creating, bearing and raising children. I believe that there is no such satisfying unit as a family. Discussions about birth, pregnancy, childhood, schooling and adolescence must surely form a large proportion of day-to-day communication amongst adults. There are few subjects so beset with old wives' tales. This book is designed to help you enjoy your children and your family life by removing, or at least putting in proportion, the instant worries that present themselves daily.

During my times as attendant obstetrician, hospital paediatrician, and clinic advisory doctor, I have been struck repeatedly by the continuing ignorance of basic facts about birth, pregnancy and childhood. If parents could pull from their bookshelves a small, practical and easily referable manual, I feel that many of those worries which become mountains might well remain molehills. I do hope this book will answer what I believe to be a very pressing need.

We do not have total control over our offspring, but at every stage we can certainly influence their development profoundly. Indeed the art of part ignoring, part guiding, and part obstructing can be fun. I have noticed with alarm in recent years, increasing despondency creeping into this whole subject. There is a feeling that we are beaten before we start; that whatever we do, the mammoth task ahead is too much and that even if our physical energy is equal to the task, our emotional and psychological approach is bound to be inadequate.

Introspection beyond a certain point, I think, is probably

7

deleterious. It is possible to delve too far into our psychological approach to our children. It is possible to get completely bogged down in rationales and theories. It is possible to forget to enjoy our children and their procreation, and the tremendous challenge that they present.

I do not believe that there is an answer to every childhood aberration. The universal law of cussedness applies to our progeny more surely than it applies anywhere else. When we look for the solution to our child's every whim in our own behaviour or attitudes, then we are in danger of letting the general become master of the individual. Not only will we fail, but we will also lose our sense of proportion and, incidentally, almost certainly our humour too.

You cannot always be the controlled, objective, cool person that you think you ought to be. The image of the ideal parent as drawn by collective advice and judgement of press, other media, public and private conscience, is not attainable. And I have no doubt that the occasional sharp rebuke by tongue or hand is not only wise but vital. But, shout at every irritating habit of your eighteen month old, or spank your toddler every time he strays out of view in an effort to enlarge his territory, and your authority and ability to discipline and even to teach will rapidly fade.

I think the most important single fact to remember when training your child is that you have to establish the pattern of day to day life for him. He needs a routine. In its earliest form he needs to learn the difference between night and day. As he grows there need to be things that always earn a reward. And similarly, later on, there need to be things that invariably cause displeasure. If you vary the response to a given stimulus your child will become confused. If he becomes confused he will become disobedient. And here you must learn to differentiate between deliberate naughtiness and the ordinary disobedience of the exploratory stage. Do not punish the latter, just the former. Finally, the child with sufficient scope to explore, both

8

mentally and physically, is much less trouble and infinitely more interesting than the frustrated, confused one.

There is no family, no father or mother who does not experience worry. Anyone who denies this is either deliberately not telling the truth, or cannot recognise the truth. Our success depends to a large extent on our attitudes to the problems which all of us face and less to the problems themselves. There is no getting away from the fact that it is hard work. There is no denying that to achieve a good family compromise, some of our own individual activities must for a while take second place.

The family who denies that the coming of children makes a difference, that they must not be allowed to rule your life, is wrong. They do make a difference; particularly on mobility and holidays, and the ease of taking instant enjoyment. But they should certainly not stop either your own special hobby or the shared evenings and outings with your spouse. If you used to enjoy a weekly trip to the cinema, you should continue this after the first week or two and when you have made adequate baby-sitting arrangements. Being a family person is certainly a more selfless existence than being alone. But the rewards are numerous. And they are to be had for such a very short time.

This book, therefore, is designed to encourage parents and prospective parents. I have arranged the facts that you will need to have at your fingertips so that they are readily available. I know the difficulties and I know the frustrations. Sometimes there is no easy answer. But certainly no good comes of restless pacings, sleepless nights and family feuds. And always remember that anxiety takes us all in different ways. What makes mother weep may well make father short-tempered. You may well be on the same side.

May I finally point out that it is the parents' job to help their children achieve independence and a useful maturity. That is all. It is not possible to ordain at what level or in what field that may be. But it is also the duty of parents to remain interesting individuals in their own right. Do not completely submerge

9

yourselves. Retain your interests; at times you will need the refuge of your own life to recover from the rigors and delights of child rearing.

Facts on Birth and Population

1 For the first time this year the number of babies being born (the birth rate), has actually fallen.

2 The size of the family unit is becoming smaller. It is comparatively rare to find a family with four children now. The accepted norm is now two or three. When families of six or eight were the rule, the survival rate of these children was, of course, much lower. But increased survival rate today still does not alter the dramatic decrease in the birth rate.

3 Added to this is the slowly increasing age of the average primip—that is the age at which you have your first baby. Many couples are leaving it much later to start their families. Here one has to weigh up the psychological advantages of the older primip against the physical advantages of the younger primip. Personally, I feel that these balance out to the mid-twenties for the average woman. But as in all things that come into the scope of this book, this is an intensely individual situation and must be discussed and decided individually.

4 I believe that families should be planned to a certain extent, but not too meticulously. There is certainly a danger in a plan which is so definite that mistakes—which can happen—might well cause major unhappiness.

This is even more important when husband and wife are not entirely in agreement. Do not be dogmatic early on in marriage about these subjects. So many of us find that our views change after a few years. And of course our circumstances change too. I think it is most important to remain flexible and such a pity to let this particular subject be a cause of family quarrels.

PART ONE

PREGNANCY

Conception

Assuming the average menstrual cycle to be twenty-eight days, ovulation takes place fourteen days after the first day of the period. Conception is most likely two days either side of this date which is often marked by a slight rise in temperature. Conception, however, may occur at any time; there is no absolutely 'safe period' when conception cannot take place, but it is more likely to be successful around ovulation. Theories about the relationship of the time interval between intercourse and ovulation, and the sex of the child, are probably valid. But I believe that a conception which is approached too scientifically is often not successful. There is no doubt that a large element of chance remains.

Failures of Conception

This is an enormously important and vital subject to many people. It cannot be comprehensively covered within the scope of this book. The points below might well be helpful, but I would stress that there is expert advice available through a general practitioner and you should not hesitate to seek it.

1 There is no doubt that excessive tension and anxiety are an important cause of failure to conceive. And in spite of the fact that this sounds so simple, it must be the most difficult thing to abolish. The one piece of advice that I would offer here is to remember that lovemaking is meant to be enjoyed for its own sake and should not only be done in a frantic and too-studied effort to conceive.

2 Similarly, although some techniques in lovemaking are undoubtedly more likely to result in conception, it is quite wrong to be uncomfortable or to subject your partner to discomfort, again simply in a frantic effort to conceive. However, the longer the sperm stay in the vagina the greater the likelihood of conception, and again, the more adequate the penetration the greater the likelihood of conception. Many couples find that

13

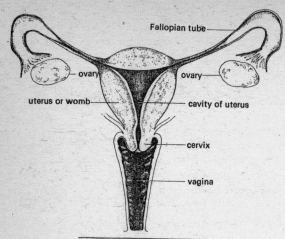

The female genital organs

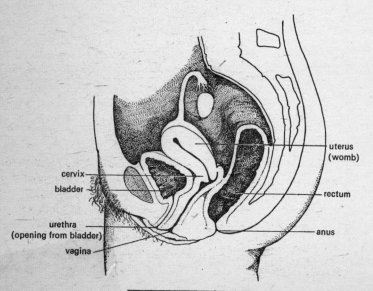

Female pelvis – from the side

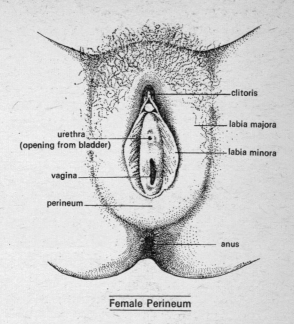

clitoris

labia majora

labia minora

urethra
(opening from bladder)

vagina

perineum

anus

Female Perineum

the front to front approach, with the women's knees drawn
well up, ensures the best penetration. Afterwards, keeping the
knees well drawn up either on your side or on your back, and if
possible with your hips higher than your stomach, will ensure
that the sperm remain high in the vagina for as long as possible.

3 Anaemia, general debility, or frank illness, especially in
the female can cause failure to conceive. It is well worth having
a general check-up.

4 And alongside these causes cannot be forgotten any actual abnormalities of the male or female sex organs. These are rare but they do occur. Remember always that it is wise for both husband and wife to have a check-up and unfair to expect one to do so and not the other.

5 Finally it must be said that women who have been on the pill do sometimes take longer to conceive than those who have not. This is one very important consideration for those wishing to start a family later. This delay in conception does not necessarily bear any correlation to the length of time that you have been on the pill. However, I would suggest that if the choice of contraceptive is the pill, and if it is important that you do have a family later on, it is wise to have a rest from the pill periodically, if you have to remain on it for a considerable length of time.

Tests for Pregnancy

1 Naturally the most obvious sign that you are pregnant is that your periods cease. But this is not always so. It is possible to have a period after you have actually conceived, although this is often an abnormally scanty one.

2 Along with the absence of the expected period, any or none of the 'early signs' listed below may appear.

3 Laboratory tests may be carried out after six weeks. That is, six weeks after the first day of the last period. These tests depend upon the presence in the urine of a certain hormone. A positive result at six weeks is conclusive. A negative result may not be so, and in the absence of menstruation, the test should be repeated weekly or fortnightly.

Early Signs and Symptoms of Pregnancy

1 Amenorrhoea is the absence of periods. Your normal blood loss does not occur and any, all, or none of the following signs may follow. Do rest assured that whereas it is perfectly

16

normal to have a certain number of these symptoms, it is not vital to have any for a successful pregnancy.

2 Breast enlargement, however, almost always occurs. It is likely to be more noticeable with a first baby and is certainly likely to be more uncomfortable with a first baby. Most commonly the sides of the breasts feel full; the whole breast feels 'tingly' and may even be actually sore. Extra little 'knobs' may appear around the nipples and the nipples themselves may irritate intensely. All the later breast changes will be found further on in the book under a separate heading.

3 Increased frequency of passing water is a very common, and often very early, symptom. But pain or burning on passing water is not normal and it is quite possible that these may be a symptom of a water infection. Urinary infection is very common in pregnancy, but, nevertheless, must be treated promptly. Frequency uncomplicated by infection often seems to be worse at night, and it is worthwhile experimenting with different ways of lying in bed. This may relieve the pressure on the bladder and thereby help the frequency. However, this can remain a truly annoying problem for some mothers throughout their pregnancy.

4 Nausea and actual vomiting are, unfortunately, very common indeed. The symptoms can vary in intensity from vague nausea in association with specific stimuli, to an intense and continuing nausea with actual vomiting for no apparent cause. 'Morning sickness' is the name frequently given to this symptom but it often does persist into the day, and indeed may even be worse in the evening. These symptoms generally start at about six to eight weeks from the first day of the last period and may indeed be the presenting symptom of pregnancy; but they usually disappear at about sixteen weeks or four months.

There is no concrete evidence of what causes the nausea of pregnancy, but there are certain things that make it worse and, I believe, some that can make it very much better. It is sometimes asserted that nausea and vomiting only occur if the

17

pregnancy is unwelcome. This is absolutely untrue. But if there are difficulties surrounding the pregnancy, any of its symptoms, including nausea, may be aggravated.

I am quite sure that hypoglycaemia, or a lowering of the blood-sugar level, is a causative factor in the vomiting of pregnancy; and I have frequently found that taking glucose or a sweet drink or even eating a biscuit can help. A cup of sweet tea before getting up can also make things better. This is not a licence to eat continuously, but it is a reminder to eat regularly.

Finally, being sick on an empty stomach is most unpleasant and very hard work, so drink a cup of warm tea anyway before getting up. That way, if you are going to be sick, it is relatively painless.

These symptoms are common and will end. I feel very strongly that it is foolish to take any medication at all during the early months of pregnancy and most of us can get through without recourse to tablets.

5 Other dietary problems include the common 'longings' for particular foods. There is no reason why these cannot be indulged unless the food itself is harmful. A desire to eat fruit should definitely be encouraged, whereas one for clotted cream should not. Some of these desires are very strange. Peppermint is often desired to the extent of eating the toothpaste rather than cleaning one's teeth with it!

Flatulence often increases in early pregnancy. There is little that will help this specifically except general hints about eating small meals often, and, again, taking a glucose tablet or barley sugar.

6 Constipation often occurs and, if not treated, can be a cause of major problems after delivery. Minor adjustments to diet may well be all that is required; for instance, just increasing the fruit or vegetable intake; but if stronger measures are needed, do not hesitate. It is such a nuisance to have chronic constipation, and this can also aggravate other conditions, such as piles. Your clinic or doctor will supply mild laxatives if a

change in diet is not sufficient, and there is absolutely no harm in using suppositories. It is not necessary to have your bowels open more than usual during your pregnancy, enough just to maintain your usual daily pattern.

7   Vaginal discharge of one sort or another is virtually always present during pregnancy. The loss of a small volume of clear or milky white fluid—that is a slight increase in the normal vaginal secretion—always occurs. Very early in pregnancy the secretion changes to a very sticky fluid, although it does not increase in amount. In fact this may well be one of the earliest signs of pregnancy.

However, the discharge should not be yellow, frothy, smelly, or in any way offensive. If it is any of these things it may well be that a mild infection is present. If so, this should be treated promptly.

8   Nose bleeds can occur in early pregnancy and I have even known this to be the very earliest sign of pregnancy. They nearly always stop after the first three months.

9   The skin undergoes small but definite changes which can certainly worry if they are not expected. The so-called mask of pregnancy is a brown discoloration of the face which may be confined to the bridge of the nose and the cheek bones, or may be more widespread to look almost like sunburn. Small red spots may also appear, especially on the face and hands. The nipples become much darker—the darker the skin type, the deeper brown they become, so that the nipples of a fair-skinned, fair-haired person may only go pale brown whereas those of a dark-haired, dark-skinned person may become almost black. Along with these changes, a dark line often appears between the umbilicus and the pubis, and moles or other birth marks frequently become darker in colour.

Diet in Pregnancy

As at all times in life the most important thing about diet is not

19

so much what it contains as the balance between the constituent parts; that is protein, fat and carbohydrate.

In many people the appetite increases; certainly mine does. Although I would not support the maxim of eating for two, I would urge most strongly that one should eat enough.

Here we come to balance. On the whole the volume of protein that you eat may be increased without harm. On the other hand, a vast increase in carbohydrate is wrong. So increase the volume of meat, fish, eggs and cheese that you eat, but resist the impulse to indulge in those extra cream cakes or potatoes.

It is very important to eat adequate amounts of vegetables and fruit because, besides satisfying your increased appetite, they will also help to counteract that most annoying of symptoms, constipation.

The average weight gain of a pregnant woman is $1\frac{1}{2}$–2 stone (9·5–12·7 kilos), but there are many women who put on less than that and some who put on more. A weight gain of less than 1 stone is definitely too little, unless, of course, you start off grossly overweight. Under these circumstances your diet becomes very important indeed and you should go through it fully with your doctor. A weight gain of more than $2\frac{1}{2}$ stone is too much and, although it may do the baby no harm, you will find it difficult to lose the surplus weight after it is born.

I do adhere to the advice that a pint of milk a day is very good. The extra vitamins that your clinic will give you are important at a time when your own health is so vital.

There are no real taboos in diet, except eating too much of any one thing. And food fads may be indulged provided they fall within the above criteria.

Smoking and Alcohol

There is no reason why alcohol may not be taken and enjoyed provided that it is in moderation. It is in fact important to remain socially normal and not to treat oneself as an invalid.

I would, however, stress that spirits should be taken with water and that to drink for drinking's sake is unwise. To get drunk would be positively irresponsible.

Smoking, however, is a different story. There can be no doubt about it. You should not smoke when you are pregnant. There can be little justification for smoking when not pregnant and absolutely none when you are.

Similarly there is no doubt that smoking during pregnancy causes a reduction in the birth weight of the child. Small and premature babies are more prone to the respiratory distress syndrome and other problems of the newborn baby (see below). Respiratory distress can kill.

Here the inevitable question arises as to whether the occasional cigarette after meals will harm the baby. It is dangerous, although probably accurate, to say no; because all too often the occasional cigarette turns into the regular one. However if it is impossible for you to stop smoking altogether, then a reduction in the number that you smoke must be the next best thing.

Sleep and Rest

In the early stages of pregnancy there should be little problem with sleeping, and normal hours of going to bed need not be altered. However, it is foolish to get overtired, and if you feel tired then you should go to bed earlier. It is unwise to have very late nights other than in exceptional circumstances, and long and arduous journeys are best avoided if possible. Later on in pregnancy sleep can become quite a problem, particularly for those who customarily sleep on their stomachs. There is no doubt that you have to learn to sleep on your back or your side. The movements of the baby will certainly disturb you late in pregnancy; they can be extraordinarily violent and, unfortunately, babies often seem more active at night than during the day.

Strangely the lack of actual sleep does not necessarily make you feel very tired and it is certainly a mistake to get up the next morning determined that you are 'done in'. You should not take sleeping tablets unless they are specifically ordered by your doctor, and this will not usually be done unless you have a slightly raised blood pressure or another medical condition that requires you to take them. In a way, this getting used to less sleep late in pregnancy prepares you for the first few weeks of your baby's life when you will need to give him four-hourly feeds, including one in the middle of the night.

Afternoon rests are a nice idea but not always practical if you have other children. However, it is sensible to try to have a 'sitting down' supervisory period, morning and afternoon, during mid and late pregnancy. If you are lucky enough to be a primip, that is a first-time mother, then make the most of it and enjoy a rest period after lunch. And this means a rest period on your bed, lying flat—so much better than a rest period in a chair. Sitting down takes little pressure off your feet and legs which is at least half the idea. So please rest on your bed and not beside it.

Exercise and Sex

This is one of those areas in which old wives' tales abound.

A normal amount of exercise is very important and walking is an excellent way to achieve it, but it is not necessary to slog ten miles a day. The idea is to keep as fit as you were before you were pregnant and not to start exercising suddenly because you become pregnant. Lifting heavy weights is not to be encouraged, not so much because of the weight, but more because of the bending that is generally involved. Incidentally, it is worthwhile practising bending at the knees while keeping a straight back. This way of bending should be continued for some time after your baby has been born because the bones and muscles of the back have undergone a lot of strain and should be guarded until they are completely recovered. Backache is such a common complaint after pregnancy and this is certainly one way in which you can guard against it.

Swimming, as for most conditions of the human body, is excellent exercise, but should not be indulged in too violently. Horse riding is probably the least sensible form of exercise during pregnancy. Certainly, any form of jumping or cross-country riding should not be done.

Now we have to consider sex. For this purpose let us divide the pregnancy into three sections.

During the first three months it is sensible to be restrained in your lovemaking. It is unlikely that gentle intercourse during a normal pregnancy will cause a miscarriage, but it is wise not to be too wild. If you have had an early miscarriage before, then definitely intercourse should be avoided, once, of course, you know that you are pregnant.

During the second three months, intercourse is perfectly possible and often very desirable. There is no need to abstain unless specifically told to by your doctor.

During the last three months it becomes more a question of personal taste and positioning rather than right or wrong. Most pregnant women continue to feel like lovemaking and their husbands too. But there is no doubt that the increasing size of the stomach makes the conventional positions of intercourse very difficult. However, if lovemaking can be achieved to the satisfaction of both partners, and without any pain or discomfort to the wife, there is absolutely no reason why it should not continue to be enjoyed. Intercourse can be perfectly satisfactory in different positions; for instance, the woman facing away from her husband and lying relaxed on her side. There is no strain on her or her baby in this position and both partners may continue to enjoy one another throughout the pregnancy. One word of warning however; if it is at all uncomfortable for the woman, intercourse should be stopped.

Medicines and Drugs

Generally speaking, the answer to what you can or cannot take safely during pregnancy, is to take nothing at all. This is one of the few things that you can do to positively help your child. You can, for example, put up with the nausea of early pregnancy. You can put up with the interrupted sleep of late pregnancy. You can modify your diet to avoid constipation.

This all sounds very hard-hearted and, as with all rules, there are always exceptions. There are, of course, times when medicines can be positively beneficial, for instance in the treatment of a urinary infection. But I would emphasise that you should not take any tablets during pregnancy lightly, and never without your doctor's express advice.

This, of course, does not apply to the vitamins and iron tablets that your antenatal clinic will give you. These will, of course, actually help the baby.

Breasts

The changes in her breasts are often the most obvious sign of all to the woman, apart, of course, from her enlarging abdomen.

The changes start with a simple feeling of fullness which then progresses to an actual enlargement. The breast may feel 'tingly' and quite uncomfortable at the sides, right under the armpits. It is in this area that you first notice the need for a new bra. All that is required is reasonable support for the enlarging breast and the only rule to remember is not to have the bra too tight. This having been said however, you can often 'make do' during the early part of pregnancy and reserve the new-bra buying until half way through. You may even be able to borrow temporarily from friends. The only rule to remember is that your breasts must be comfortable. If you are going to feed your baby yourself it will be necessary to buy good feeding bras for this purpose.

If you are planning to breast-feed your baby, it is most important that your nipples are properly prepared during pregnancy. If your nipples are small, or inverted, then they may be prepared for feeding by using nipple shields. It is such a shame when you are unable to breast-feed purely because of the lack of a little simple preparation. Unfortunately, it is sometimes necessary to 'nag' for the kind of help that you need, although most clinics are very helpful.

As pregnancy proceeds, the nipple and the surrounding areola change colour, becoming darker. Also, extra little knobs or swellings grow around the nipple. Many people experience a little discharge from the nipple which, although not sufficient to be noticed in itself, may cause crusting to appear. It is unusual for there to be any milk production before birth if you are a primip, but for those mothers expecting second or third babies it is quite common.

Those people who get stretch marks on the stomach and thighs during pregnancy, often get smaller stretch marks on the breasts.

Many women ask whether breast-feeding will alter the shape and size of their breasts after it is stopped. The answer is that, usually, the breast size decreases after feeding, although the breasts may remain just as firm. As usual there are exceptions to the rule, but in the vast majority of cases the breasts will become a little smaller. This is because, in order to feed adequately, much of the fatty tissue in the breast is replaced by milk ducts and when those milk ducts become empty, when feeding has finished, the volume of the breast will obviously be less.

Stretch Marks and the Skin

Who will get stretch marks? There is no easy answer. On the whole fairer, drier skin is more likely to get them than darker, oilier skin. But there is no hard and fast rule. Certainly if you

25

got stretch marks while you were on the pill you will get them when you are pregnant.

You cannot on the whole prevent them. But I believe that you can make them not so bad. Many people use baby oil over the abdomen as it enlarges, but I have found that bath oil in the bath itself seems to have the same result and is certainly a great deal less trouble. The object is to try and make the skin more elastic.

As for treating the stretch marks after delivery, the single most important thing is to lose the excess weight as quickly as possible and to restore the tone to the muscles of your stomach wall. Swimming, particularly, is an excellent toning-up exercise. There is no real substitute for natural toning-up of the skin but the practice of many health clinics in using 'Slendertone' does seem to have some good results.

As a final comment, there is no doubt that a good tan covers up a lot of the smaller stretch marks, so do not throw away your bikini because you have been unfortunate enough to get them.

Other skin changes have already been dealt with. They do not necessarily occur, although the changes in the nipple colour are fairly constant. And, again, many of them, except those in the nipple, will often disappear when the pregnancy is over. The changes are much more pronounced in the darker-skinned individual and none of them will do any harm at all.

Vaginal Discharge

A small amount of clear or slightly milky fluid is absolutely normal. The actual amount varies from person to person. In pregnancy this volume nearly always increases. However, if this discharge becomes yellow or greenish-yellow, or becomes irritating, then it is possible that there is a vaginal infection. These mild vaginal infections are fairly common anyway, becoming more so on the pill, and very common indeed during pregnancy. They should be treated promptly and completely.

Any blood-staining in the discharge or actual blood loss is not normal and should be reported and investigated. As vaginal discharge does have this increased incidence, the daily bath at this time becomes even more important. There is no contra-indication to frequent baths, but these should not be too hot, as there is an increased tendency to fainting anyway in pregnancy and very hot baths can aggravate this tendency.

Care of Hair, Nails and Teeth

On the whole the condition of most peoples' hair improves during pregnancy. All it requires is the usual washing routine. Occasionally, however, hair falls out and sometimes in quite alarming quantities. This need not be a cause for concern provided there is no scalp disease. It will resolve itself spontaneously and needs no treatment.

Sometimes the condition of the nails also deteriorates. This can be due to lack of calcium in the diet and may be helped by increasing your intake of milk.

Care of the teeth is also very important and it is worthwhile mentioning that dental care is free to expectant mothers. Teeth certainly seem to decay more readily during pregnancy and gums bleed more often. So, as a routine, go and see your dentist at the beginning of your pregnancy.

Bowels and Haemorrhoids

As has already been mentioned, it is extremely common for the expectant mother to tend to become more constipated and very important to prevent this as it can be quite a nuisance, not only during pregnancy, but also during delivery and after the baby is born.

Constipation, of course, predisposes to haemorrhoids which can also become a major problem. Haemorrhoids are varicose veins of the anus and are caused by pressure above the veins. Hence, they are common in any pregnancy and even more so in one that is complicated by constipation. There is no doubt that in the majority of cases constipation may be prevented, and even cured, by proper and rigorous attention to diet. The obvious thing to do is to increase your intake of fruit and vegetables. Changing to wholemeal bread may be all that is required. If it is not possible for you to cure your own constipation by attention to diet, then you must get expert help.

Maternity Clothes

In the early weeks of pregnancy there is no need, and indeed it is foolish, to go out and spend a lot of money on maternity clothes. However, it is important to wear things that are comfortable and certainly anything that is tight around the waist will not improve your nausea, while anything tight across the bust will be most uncomfortable.

Later on, to invest in a really capacious pair of slacks is a great investment, as the availability of very pretty smocks to go over them is almost unlimited. I have found that outsize tights worn back to front are a splendid fit even for the very largest stomach and are very much cheaper than tights designed especially for the pregnant woman.

Bra support I have dealt with in the previous section on the care of the breasts.

Towards the end of pregnancy, I believe that there is no greater boost to the morale than to go out and buy at least one really attractive outfit. By the time you are about seven months pregnant you will be almost as large as you are going to get and it is important for your well being that you do keep your morale up. The last two months often seem to last for ever especially if you have to wear the same clothes every day. So, if you can afford it, do your spending later rather than earlier.

Lastly, shoes should be worn for comfort, but there is no reason why they should not also be fashionable. However, excessively high heels might well cause you to fall over—your centre of gravity changes while you are pregnant, with the increasing weight out at the front and makes it more difficult to balance. Slightly flatter shoes are much safer and often you will find them more comfortable too. Also, even in the most normal pregnancy, there is a slight degree of ankle swelling and shoes must cater for this.

Illness During Pregnancy

It is obviously wise to remain as healthy as possible during your pregnancy. It is sensible, therefore, to avoid direct contact with anyone who is suffering from an infectious disease. This is particularly important in early pregnancy, not only because this is the time when all the baby's organs are being formed, but because a sudden high temperature can occasionally precipitate a miscarriage.

The specific infection which causes most anxiety in pregnancy is rubella, or German measles. So important is this that all secondary-school children are now being offered immunisation against it, as a precaution for the child bearing years ahead, and those women who have not had German measles are offered immunisation after the birth of their first baby. Rubella can cause actual congenital abnormalities of hearing, sight, heart, and brain and any contact with someone who has got rubella should be avoided or reported. It is possible to take blood tests to tell whether or not a patient has had rubella and a certain amount of immunological help can be offered in the case of clinical infection. But there remain a few cases where a severe infection of rubella, between the sixth and tenth week, may be a valid reason for a therapeutic abortion.

The other important specific infection which must be watched for during pregnancy is, of course, venereal disease and, in particular, syphilis. All antenatal clinics will, as routine, test for this at your first visit. Any subsequent possible infection should be reported immediately.

Changes in Mid-Pregnancy

As pregnancy advances further, somewhat smaller but definite changes take place in the body. Some of these can be quite worrying if they are not expected.

1   Firstly the baby continues to grow and the shape and size of the abdomen with it. By the doctor, the enlarging womb can

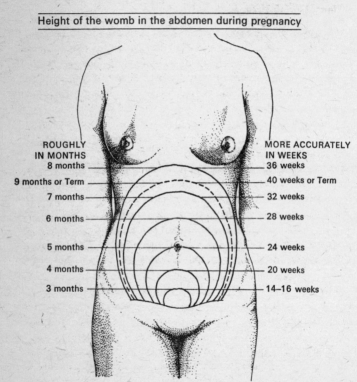

Height of the womb in the abdomen during pregnancy

ROUGHLY IN MONTHS	MORE ACCURATELY IN WEEKS
8 months	36 weeks
9 months or Term	40 weeks or Term
7 months	32 weeks
6 months	28 weeks
5 months	24 weeks
4 months	20 weeks
3 months	14–16 weeks

The height of the fundus (or top) of the uterus falls in the last month as the head of the baby goes down into the pelvis be felt, first, in the abdomen, after the third month. Before that it is only felt in the pelvis. By the fifth month the enlarging uterus has reached the level of the umbilicus and it then continues to rise up the abdomen until it is felt right under the ribs where it can become very uncomfortable. At about the eighth month, however, particularly in a first baby, the baby's head drops down into the pelvis, preparing for birth, and the pressure under the ribs suddenly becomes much less.

There is a vast variety of stomach 'shapes' and there is no truth in the statement that 'all out in front' means one sex and 'all out at the sides' means another. Certain shapes of the pelvic bones predispose the baby towards lying with its back facing backwards, instead of the slightly more usual position of the back facing forwards. The former position will cause a flat top to the abdomen.

Second babies are nearly always carried further forwards because the muscles of the abdominal wall 'give' quicker during a second pregnancy.

The shape of the abdomen does not tell you the sex of your child. Indeed, nothing will for certain. However, I do believe that in many people a male pregnancy is different from a female pregnancy and the experienced mother may well be able to tell you what sex of child she will have. Personally I feel that too much speculation in this direction is often very harmful and as far as possible it is much more sensible to keep an open mind as to the sex of your unborn child.

2   Any time from the sixteenth week onwards you will begin to feel the baby move. Mothers having a second or subsequent baby will, on the whole, feel movements earlier while those having a first baby may well have to wait until twenty or twenty-two weeks (the fifth month). Partly, of course, this is because the experienced mother knows what to expect. The earliest movements feel like a fluttering butterfly low in your stomach; they are very slight at first, and then become progressively stronger.

At the same time as this, the examining doctor can hear the

baby's heart beating. Obviously if the heart can be heard, it is conclusive proof that the baby has quickened, but the converse is not true. If at this early stage the heartbeat cannot be heard then it does not mean that all is not well. If you are having twins it is occasionally possible to hear two individual heartbeats because they are beating at different rates, but this is not always the case and no reliance can be placed on it. It is possible to magnify the sound of the heartbeat with a machine and if you are in hospital at any time you may be lucky enough to hear your baby's heartbeat very clearly. However, I must stress that this is not a routine procedure.

3 At about the sixth or seventh month the enlarging baby can cause quite a change in breathing. The baby, particularly if it is a breech, is pushing up under the ribs and may be very uncomfortable. You can help this quite considerably by always sitting up straight. You should by this time have learnt to breathe with your chest-wall more than with your stomach muscles and increasing your ability to do this will greatly help during delivery. Just before delivery, and possibly up to a month before, the breathing suddenly becomes easier again as the baby goes down into the pelvis and positions itself for going down the birth canal. Now uncomfortable pressure may be felt down in the pelvis, and in women who have had several babies this can be very uncomfortable indeed.

4 In addition to the frequency of passing water, which may occur throughout pregnancy, at these later stages actual leakage of water is very common, particularly at times of stress such as coughing or sneezing.

5 Inevitably, at this stage, the question of viability comes up. 'When is the baby mature enough to live?' There is no easy answer. At present the law states that the dividing line is twenty-eight weeks. The loss of a foetus before that time is termed a miscarriage and after that date a stillbirth. But, at the time of writing, the law is under review and may well be altered. Certainly there have been many accounts of more premature

32

foetuses surviving, and there are also countless numbers of foetuses, older than twenty-eight weeks, who have been too imma-
ture to survive. Much religious feeling points to actual conception
being the beginning of life, but in no sense can a foetus be
termed viable (ie capable of independent existence) at that
stage. There will always have to be an arbitrary dividing line
and it will always continue to be a very vexed and emotive
subject.

6   Throughout middle pregnancy, the uterus may be seen to
contract periodically. These are not labour contractions and are,
on the whole, painless, although they may be an odd enough
feeling to be termed very uncomfortable. During late pregnancy,
these contractions do most definitely become painful in some
women, although they are different from labour pains. They
may be precipitated by sudden, or unduly strenuous, exercise
and anything that does cause them is probably better avoided.
However, they may also occur quite spontaneously while at rest
and, just as spontaneously, disappear. Real contractions, at the
onset of labour, are usually felt lower in the abdomen and in the
back, and will also increase in intensity and frequency quite
steadily.

Possible Procedures in Mid-Pregnancy

During the course of your pregnancy it may be necessary for
you to undergo a more specialised form of investigation, so that
your attendant doctors may decide definitely, for example,
whether you are expecting twins, or if the baby is upside down
(ie a breech). Some of these procedures are explained briefly
below as most of the worrying that you do is because you
neither know nor understand what is going on. None of them is
as serious as is often imagined.

1   X-ray used to be the only way to tell definitely the
occurrence and position of twins. It could also give a reasonably
accurate assessment of maturity. But there is no doubt that the

use of X-rays, particularly in early pregnancy, does carry a health risk to the baby, and in many hospitals the use of ultrasound (see below) has superseded X-ray diagnosis. However, in later pregnancy, and occasionally during labour itself, an X-ray will give a quick and easy view of the situation with absolutely no risk to the baby.

2 Version, again, is less commonly practised now than it used to be. It is somewhat easier to deliver a baby head first than feet first, simply because the head acts as a more effective opener of the birth canal. Therefore, if a baby is in the breech position, many practitioners will attempt to turn it round at about the thirty-second–thirty-fourth week (seventh–eighth month), and therefore encourage the head to engage in the pelvis. This simple manoeuvre involves the mother lying on a bed, relaxed, occasionally with the help of some medicine, while the doctor gently manipulates the baby round. This may feel strange but it certainly does not hurt.

3 Ultrasound is the new method by which we see many of the things that would formerly have been discovered by X-ray. There is absolutely no pain or discomfort involved, except that of lying on a hard bed for a length of time! This procedure produces a picture of the baby in the womb which can be measured to tell the baby's size, maturity and orientation most accurately. It can, of course, also show whether there are one, two, or three babies. And it can also define accurately where the afterbirth or placenta is, to make sure that it is not in front of the baby's head where it will proceed down the birth canal. While making of this very accurate diagnosis there is no harm at all to the baby and no risk at all to the mother.

4 Amniocentesis is the name given to the taking off of a small quantity of the fluid surrounding the baby in the womb. From an examination of this fluid and the cells contained in it, it is possible to find out whether the baby has certain types of inherited diseases. Currently its use is in the diagnosis of such disorders as spina bifida. The procedure does carry a very

slight risk and it is therefore reserved for those people who have a particular and special problem and who run a high risk of having an abnormal baby. Apart from this limitation there is another, in that the procedure is not done in all hospitals or clinics.

5 Finally there are special problems associated with those mothers who have rhesus incompatibility. Thankfully this, which used to be such a common and serious complication of pregnancy, has been virtually eliminated by the use of the anti-D factor which is effective in stopping rhesus incompatibility in all later pregnancies, provided no antibodies are produced during the first pregnancy. There remains a small minority of mothers, having a second or subsequent baby, where it is still a problem. The special procedures of transfusion and exchange transfusion in the womb are still occasionally necessary.

Some Common Disorders of Pregnancy

1 Early miscarriage or abortion (this term is the official medical one and does not imply interference) remains the most common of all the things that can go wrong after conception. In fact, one in five conceptions will end in miscarriage, although many of these are so slight that they are taken as 'late periods'. In most cases the reason for this very early miscarriage will be unproven, but there is no doubt that a large proportion will be due to ovum (egg) abnormality or hormone insufficiency and therefore quite beyond anyone's control. If, in fact, the woman suffers from early repeated miscarriages, it is likely that hormone deficiency is the reason and injections of added hormones may well be necessary. If a miscarriage is threatened, bedrest is often advisable because the mother feels tired or unwell, but I'm afraid that this will very rarely, if at all, have any effect on whether the foetus is lost or not.

2 There is a small but very significant number of miscarriages which are due to the inability of the cervix (the neck

35

of the womb) to hold the growing foetus inside. Miscarriages in these cases are usually between the third and fifth month. The condition is known as cervical incompetence and may be prevented in a subsequent pregnancy by stitching up the neck of the womb for the duration of the pregnancy and undoing the stitch when delivery is imminent.

3 The common infectious disorders of pregnancy have already been discussed. I mention them again, briefly, however, because they are so important. Vaginal infection, particularly thrush (monilia), remains the most important. Second to this comes urinary tract infection which must be treated promptly.

4 Following on from a discussion of urinary tract infection comes the most important and, incidentally, the commonest of all the disorders associated with pregnancy. This is toxaemia of pregnancy, having a triad of symptoms: (a) raised blood pressure; (b) protein in the urine, and (c) swelling of the soft tissues, of the ankles and hands in particular. This swelling is called oedema. It is necessary for two of these symptoms to be present to make a diagnosis of toxaemia. This is a particularly important thing to say because nearly all women experience some amount of oedema or swelling, even if it is only enough to make a wedding ring a little tighter. This does not mean that they have toxaemia. Although the diagnosis of toxaemia is fairly clear cut, the cause remains obscure—there are various theories, but nobody yet knows for certain.

The importance of toxaemia is in its effect primarily on the baby, and secondly on the mother, if it remains unchecked. In itself it may decrease the growth of the child, and in its secondary effect of predisposition to ante-partum haemorrhage, it may further retard that growth. If it cannot be checked then, for the sake of the health of both baby and mother, induction of labour must often be carried out early. The main treatment of toxaemia remains bedrest with slight sedation to ensure adequate rest during the day and sleeping tablets to ensure really complete rest at night. Reduction in the salt intake of the mother is also used, and sometimes other medicines as well. There is nothing more to it than that, but for the vast majority of women it is too tall an order for home. And certainly if you are surrounded by other young children it is virtually impossible to get adequate rest. However, if your doctor tells you to go home and rest, you would be well advised to do so, because if the amount of bedrest that you get is inadequate to lower your blood pressure or reduce your oedema, then you will almost certainly have to go into hospital to achieve just that.

5   Severe toxaemia may be accompanied by small losses of blood. However, this is only one of the causes of blood loss during pregnancy and any loss of blood is potentially of great importance and must be reported at once. The afterbirth or placenta may be in front of the baby's head blocking the passage through to the birth canal. Usually the afterbirth is at the side or on the top of the womb well out of the way. It is possible now by the use of ultrasound equipment, if it is available, to find out exactly where the placenta is. Even if it is situated right in the way it is of course quite possible to deliver the baby quite safely by Caesarian section.

6   Although less important in terms of morbidity than the placenta praevia discussed above, varicose veins and their special name when around the anus, haemorrhoids, are a considerable nuisance to many women. Both these conditions are due, more or less, to the increase in pressure in the pelvis due to the enlarging womb. As with so many of the symptoms of pregnancy the cure for this is as much rest as possible. In the case of varicose veins, pressure must be taken off the pelvic veins and rest must be taken on a bed, or at least with ankles and legs well up above the level of the hips. Support, in the form of elastic stockings, can relieve the ache which so often accompanies varicose veins. It will cheer up many people to know that the varicose veins of pregnancy often disappear entirely after delivery, although they will almost certainly return in a subsequent pregnancy.

Haemorrhoids have already been dealt with in the section on constipation. Never was the maxim more true than in this case, that it is better to prevent than to have to cure. However, there are a number of preparations which can help considerably if you are unfortunate enough to suffer in this way. Of primary importance is to keep the bowels open and this can be done in a variety of ways with your doctor's help. Secondly, local irritation and pain can be relieved by creams or suppositories. Whatever is prescribed for you, it is very important to keep up the treatment for a while even after everything seems to have returned to normal.

7 Excessive vomiting can occur in pregnancy and when it is so severe as to constitute an illness, it is known as hyperemesis gravidarum. I believe, however, except in these rare cases, although the vomiting of pregnancy varies from woman to woman, the attitude and approach to that vomiting is also of great importance. In the first instance, it must be recognised that the nausea and vomiting of pregnancy is so common as to be considered normal. It is nothing to be ashamed of and in no way reflects the ability of the woman to be a mother. It is certainly not due to guilt or to an underlying desire not to be pregnant, as has been postulated in the past. However, anxiety and tension can make it worse and the most vital thing is, firstly, to accept it as normal and, secondly, to change your eating habits to suit the sickness pattern. For instance, many women find that they vomit most for three to four hours on waking and thereafter very little, if at all. Therefore, it would be sensible to drink hot sweet tea during this time and reserve the main meals for later in the day. This is for two reasons.

There is considerable evidence, I believe, for the belief that the sickness is worse if the blood-sugar level goes down. Hence sugar or glucose can help for many people. Secondly, it is very painful, particularly with an enlarging stomach, to vomit at all; and it is considerably easier to vomit a thin fluid than a large heavy meal. This sort of approach may be adopted at whatever

38

is the worst time of the day for the individual. Be objective about the situation and rest assured on two counts; one, it is not your fault and two, it will stop—usually by the fourth month, although if you are unlucky it may go on a little longer.

8 One of the tests carried out on all pregnant women is a routine urine test, and among the things that are looked for is sugar. It is possible to have sugar in the urine perfectly harmlessly, but it can also be the first sign of diabetes. There are women who, although perfectly well when not pregnant, show the early signs of diabetes when they are pregnant. If their diet is properly worked out, this can be controlled and, in fact, blood and urine tests will return to normal after the pregnancy.

9 Finally, it is quite common for pregnant women to become anaemic. This is why you are routinely given iron tablets to take. However, there are other types of anaemia and occasionally other forms of treatment are necessary.

Doctor Care During Pregnancy

The care of you and your baby will be divided between your own general practitioner, your practitioner's midwife and the maternity hospital, which may be a large one with consultants and junior doctors in attendance, or a small cottage hospital run by specialist general practitioners with consultant cover. How this care is organised may be in one of several ways.

1 You may go to hospital for all your antenatal clinics, be delivered in hospital, and have your post-natal examination there too.

2 You may be seen at the hospital antenatal clinic on some visits and be able to go to your own general practitioner for most of the others. Still, your actual delivery will be at the maternity hospital, although your post-natal examination, provided that your delivery was normal, will be with your own doctor.

3 Your GP may undertake all your antenatal care and you

may have your baby also under his care at the local, small cottage hospital.

4 Finally, all your antenatal care may be undertaken by your GP and he may also agree to let you have your baby at home.

The last arrangement is becoming increasingly uncommon and in my opinion rightly so. I believe, in common with nearly all obstetricians, that all deliveries ought to take place in hospital. This is not because hospital is the nicest place, but because if there is any difficulty with the baby, for instance breathing difficulty, all the equipment is at hand to deal with it. Similarly, if there is any last-minute difficulty from the mother's point of view, it is very distressing to have to be transferred to hospital at the last minute while in labour. However, if your first pregnancy was entirely normal in every respect and if your present pregnancy has been uneventful and your GP is willing to deliver you at home, and if being delivered at home is of very great importance to you, then I would say go ahead. But unless the answer to all these questions is yes, then I think it is an unnecessary risk to have a baby at home.

The forty-eight hours that you would be in hospital, in the event of an uncomplicated delivery, should not be so great an upset for any existing member of the family. And, more than that, a few nights of uninterrupted sleep for the mother, and particularly a few days' respite from the demands of all the rest of the family, can prove a very valuable start for the increased demands of a new baby. Make the best arrangements that you possibly can for your husband and your children and, having done so, relax and do your best to get as much rest as possible.

As for how much of your antenatal care is undertaken by your GP and how much by the hospital, this depends mainly on your past obstetric history, ie your previous pregnancies.

A woman expecting her first baby, or a woman whose past obstetric history has been reasonably uncomplicated, will be seen at the beginning of the pregnancy at the hospital antenatal clinic, at the eighth month (thirty-six weeks) at the hospital, and then on the date that you are due and every subsequent week that your pregnancy is allowed to go over time. Your doctor will see you on every other visit and will arrange for additional hospital appointments if he feels they are necessary.

A woman who, for any reason, needs special watching will be seen more often at the hospital clinic.

These varying arrangements may sound very complicated, but they are designed so that every woman gets the greatest amount of continuity available and so that any woman needing extra specialist care can have access to it at any time. Similarly, it is designed so that those women whose pregnancy is uncomplicated and whose health remains excellent, may see their own doctor close to home and in comparative comfort without having to go to the hospital.

Wherever you go, at various stages of pregnancy, the routine at each visit tends to be the same.

1   At the booking clinic, usually at about three months, that is when you are certain that you are pregnant, the doctor who sees you will take the details of your present pregnancy, any previous pregnancies, your medical history and all your relevant family history. This is very time consuming, but really is necessary. You will then be examined including a general physical examination with blood pressure reading, an examination of your abdomen, and usually an internal examination as well. This is occasionally omitted, for instance if you have a history of recurrent miscarriage. After this, specimens of urine and blood will be taken for analysis and, finally, you will be asked to make a further appointment. This is all likely to take a long time, but be patient, it will not be so bad next time.

2   From booking clinic to about the eighth month, the routine at the antenatal clinic, whether you are seen by your GP or by a hospital doctor, is likely to be the same. You will take a urine specimen to be tested and your blood pressure will be checked.

41

Your abdomen will be examined and the doctor will also check your ankles and hands for swelling. You will generally need to see the doctor every four weeks until the seventh month, then every two weeks until the eighth month, then every week until you are delivered.

3   At the thirty-sixth week, another internal examination will be performed to make sure that the baby will pass easily through the birth passages.

4   From then on the doctor will be checking to see if at any time, for the sake of the baby or the mother, delivery should be hastened. For instance, if you have mild toxaemia and the baby seems to be a good size, it may well be considered wise to start off your labour a little early. However, if you and the baby continue to be well, then no attempt to induce you will be made until after the date you were originally given. It is unlikely that you will be allowed to go more than two weeks overdue, but this is dealt with more fully in the chapter on induction.

Help During Pregnancy

During pregnancy, as at no other time in your life, advice and help will pour in from all quarters. Some of this will be misplaced but all of it will be well meant. So bear with it, but make sure that you go to the recognised antenatal classes recommended by your midwife if you have any particular questions or worries. Even if you do not have any problems that you wish to discuss, the friendship of other women at the same stage of labour and pregnancy is very comforting to all of us. You may well find that someone you have met at the classes will be in hospital at the same time as you when you are finally ready to have the baby.

I am sure that a certain amount of preparation is of great value, but I, personally, feel that it is possible to have too much information. Many films, for instance on actual childbirth, are very distressing to some women, partly, I suspect, because they

42

are very emotional because of their pregnancy anyway, but much more because the personal involvement, which makes childbirth such a tremendous experience, is missing when you are just passively watching a film. I have endeavoured in the next part of this book to give a factual account of delivery which should help you, but I think that too graphic a film is not a good idea for most people. As to whether your husband should attend; if he has a specific worry then I think it important that he should voice it and one of the best ways to do that is either to meet the midwives at the antenatal class, or to go and meet the ward staff if this can be arranged. Some clinics run a special session for husbands and wives together and this is obviously very valuable. However, the routine antenatal clinics are usually designed for the mothers alone. And again, as with women, I believe that films are probably of little value. In fact they more often shock and alarm than instruct and calm.

1   Antenatal classes will teach you care of the breasts, pre- and post-natal exercises, how to breathe and cope better with delivery itself, and very many other aspects of pregnancy, labour and early childhood.

2   Psychoprophylaxis is the name given to just one of these forms of preparation. This is a method based on the work of the scientist Pavlov, and is the conditioning of women to cope without drugs or pain in labour. When this preparation is comprehensive then its results are excellent, but I feel that any complete method of preparation is just as good. This consists of a full understanding of the mechanics of labour, a full understanding of what will be expected of you, of how much help you will receive and the acquisition of a few learned skills that will help in all these objectives.

3   Your relatives can be, and often are, of great value and great support. Remember that mothers and mothers-in-law have had babies themselves and, although attitudes may have changed in some respects, they will understand the emotions involved. They will understand from first hand experience many

of the symptoms of pregnancy. Of even greater importance they will understand the need for rest. So if they volunteer to have your other child or children for the afternoon, accept, and enjoy your leisure. The other children will enjoy it too; waiting for a new brother or sister often seems to them to go on for ever. But remember also that pregnancy and childbirth abound with old wives' tales handed down through generations. Some of these tales can be quite frightening. If in doubt, do ask your doctor or your midwife.

Are You Ready?

Having a case ready packed for yourself and one for your husband to bring in for the baby can save several minutes of acute anxiety when the time actually comes to go into hospital. Most hospital clinics will give you a list of what to bring but if they do not you will need:

For yourself—

2 nightdresses (cotton if possible)

3 pairs of pants (these should not be worn immediately after delivery if you can help it, because the perineum will heal much more quickly if allowed to 'breathe')

1 sanitary belt

1 packet of maternity towels (these will often be provided)

1 dressing-gown

2 towels

toilet requisites, ie brush, comb, soap, flannel, toothbrush and toothpaste, etc

1 pair of slippers

bras—feeding bras if you are hoping to breast-feed

For the baby (your husband can bring this in later)—

1 Babygro

2 nappies

2 nappy pins

pram set or some kind of warm outer clothing

plastic pants

a shawl or bedclothes in a carry cot depending on how you are going to get home

I will discuss the nursery, bedclothes and baby clothing in Part Three.

PART TWO

DELIVERY

How Long is a Pregnancy?

The normal pregnancy lasts for forty weeks. Your doctor will calculate the exact date you are due by counting forward nine calendar months and then on for a further week. I find it simpler to go back just three months and then forward one week. Both of these calculations are made from the first day of your last period. For instance, if the first day of your last period was 20 August, then go backwards three months—20 May—and then forwards one week—27 May. This calculation is only completely accurate for those people who have an average menstrual cycle of twenty-eight days. If your period cycle is longer, then the expected date of delivery is later, and if your period cycle is shorter, then the expected date of delivery may be sooner. Calculation of the EDD (estimated date of delivery) may also be upset after being on the pill. It is quite possible to miss several periods after being on the pill, but still conceive during this time.

You will be further confused, however, because all the dates given to you at your antenatal clinics will be reckoned in weeks up to a total of forty weeks. The date at which, in law, a baby is said to be viable, is twenty-eight weeks, which is not seven months because each calendar month contains more than four weeks. It is more accurate to say that twenty-eight weeks is only six months. I have known these differences to cause the most amazing confusion, so if you can learn to think in weeks it will help you, and incidentally your doctor, a great deal.

Prematurity is the term used for those babies born before the estimated date of delivery. The degree of their prematurity is given in weeks, ie a thirty-seven week premature baby would be one which was born three weeks before the estimated date of delivery.

Post-mature is the name given to those babies born after the estimated date of delivery.

Both these conditions carry special difficulties and hazards and therefore it is very important, firstly, to estimate the date of delivery accurately and, secondly, to try to achieve delivery at about that date although a few days either way do no harm at all.

Normal Onset of Labour

Having waited for nine months for your baby to make its appearance, the last week or two of your pregnancy often seems an eternity. And, I am afraid, the time is often beset with false alarms. Many symptoms are hopefully hailed as signs of impending labour, but there are, in fact, very few ways in which normal labour can begin.

1   Surprisingly, the very best way that your labour can begin is by having twenty-four hours' diarrhoea. This ensures that the lower bowel is empty, leaving all the room in the pelvis for the birth passages to dilate so that your baby can be born easily. The same result is achieved artificially by giving you an enema at the onset of labour when you arrive at the hospital.

2   'The show' is the name given to a variable quantity of a bloodstained, jelly-like substance which is passed as the birth passages begin to dilate. Because the blood is mixed with a lot of mucus, the resultant colour is pink. It should not be pure, bright red blood. Any loss of pure blood must be reported immediately.

3   Backache is also very common at the onset of labour. It is generally felt very low in the back and is nagging and persistent and not altered by any change in posture.

4   The baby in the womb is surrounded by a 'bag of water'. When the baby is finally ready to be born, this bag will break. In some people it breaks very early on and is a sign of impending labour that should make you go into hospital. Occasionally the bag breaks very late in labour and may indeed have to be broken by your doctor or midwife. Whenever it breaks, it is not the slightest bit painful and you will only know that it has

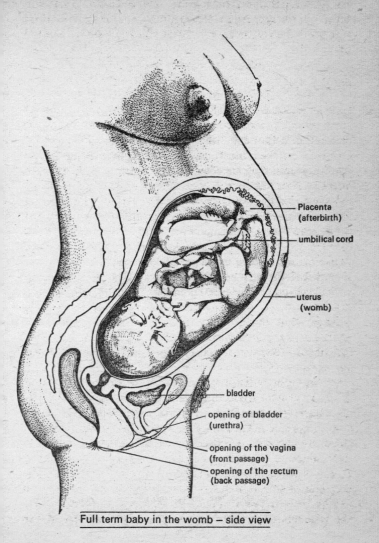

Placenta
(afterbirth)

umbilical cord

uterus
(womb)

bladder

opening of bladder
(urethra)

opening of the vagina
(front passage)

opening of the rectum
(back passage)

Full term baby in the womb – side view

happened through being soaked with the water that is released!
So do not worry if it does break. Ring the hospital if you are to
be delivered there, or your doctor if you are being delivered at
home.

5   Finally, of course, there are the pains themselves which,
in some people, are the onset of labour. In some they may
follow the show or the breaking of the waters. Whenever they
start, they come infrequently at first. They are low in your
stomach and, if you are used to them, they are just like period
pains at first. They come and go more than period pains, however, and often go into your back. Gradually they increase in
frequency until they are coming quite regularly, say, every ten
minutes or so. Although they are uncomfortable, they are by no
means unbearable at this stage, in fact, provided that the waters
have not broken, many people find that they feel better if they
continue to move around and even do some light chores. Once
they are coming quite regularly, however, it is a sign that you
should get ready to go into hospital. It is a pity to go there too
soon, because it may be a false alarm and the pains may stop
again which can be very disappointing. On the other hand, you
should try to get to hospital in a calm unflustered manner,
without an undignified dash at the last minute. If you are having
a first baby then there is not quite so much of a rush as labour
takes longer on the whole than with a second or subsequent
baby. As a general rule, once the pains are coming regularly
—every 5–10 minutes—it is wise to get to the hospital, giving
yourself time to arrive there calmly, ready for the real job
of having the baby. If you are worried as to whether to go or
not, always ring the maternity ward, the sister in charge would
much rather advise you over the telephone than have a mad
rush on her doorstep at the last minute.

Abnormal Signs at the Onset of Labour

1   Fresh bleeding is not a normal sign at the onset of labour.

It can mean that the afterbirth is blocking the passage of the baby's head down the birth canal. Bleeding should be reported and you should go into hospital.

2 If you should feel anything solid in the entrance of the vagina, particularly if the waters break suddenly and there is a lot of water lost, this may mean that the baby's head is not coming down first which is the commonest way. This again should be reported and you should go into hospital.

3 Anything else other than the signs listed above as normal should be reported and if you are in any doubt at all, ring your doctor or, preferably, the maternity hospital where you are booked in to have your baby.

Induction of Labour

It may well be that your doctor will decide it is better for you or your baby if it is delivered without waiting for you to go into labour of your own accord. From the mother's point of view this can be very disappointing, particularly if you feel that everything about having your baby should be as natural as possible. However, it really is advisable in certain circumstances and your doctor will not take the decision to 'start you off' lightly.

1 Toxaemia is one of the commonest reasons for induction. When you have toxaemia, the afterbirth, or placenta, does not continue to work as well as it might. If the toxaemia is mild, and your baby continues to grow, then your doctor may well be happy for you to continue to 'term', or forty weeks, but very unhappy for the pregnancy to continue after that date. In these circumstances, he will let you go on to term and will then plan to get you into hospital to start you off in labour. If the day that he chooses seems to be for his convenience rather than yours, then this is simply because he knows that once he has started you off he will need to be constantly at hand until you are delivered. It would be no good him starting you off on a

morning when he knew he would be in the operating theatre all day.

Of course if the toxaemia begins to get worse, and there is evidence that the baby is not going to grow any bigger inside the womb, then he may make a sudden and earlier plan to get you into hospital. Whatever way he plans it, you may rest assured that it will be in your baby's and your own interests. And at least one part of this decision is making sure that he or one of his colleagues will be at hand to deliver your baby.

2   Post-maturity is another reason for induction. It is rare for an obstetrician to let you go more than two weeks after your expected date of delivery, provided of course that the date of your last period was certain and that your periods are reasonably regular. However, this, like most rules, is sometimes broken. For instance, if your menstrual cycle is abnormally long then you may be allowed to go a little longer over your time. If, on the other hand, you tend to have large babies, the baby seems a very good size, and you have stopped putting on weight, you may be started off just a few days after your expected date. As in so many decisions in obstetrics, all the pros and cons have to be continually weighed up. Your doctor will discuss it all with you.

3   There are a number of medical reasons for induction which relate to the mother. For instance, babies being born to diabetic mothers are usually induced early and sometimes as much as four weeks early.

4   While the baby is growing in the womb, certain hormones are being passed out in the urine. By measuring the concentration of these hormones, an idea can be obtained of the rate of the baby's growth. If that growth suddenly stops, or there are other untoward signs, this may also make your doctor start you off early.

The idea in all these decisions is to achieve the safest and easiest birth for mother and baby.

Methods of Induction

1 The simplest of these is the bath and enema routine, which is still widely followed. The bath is, firstly, for the obvious reason of hygiene and, secondly, because, having just arrived in hospital, a warm bath is a reasonable way to try and relax. It has the advantage of being just a bit private, and for many women one of the most unnerving things about having a baby is the sudden and complete publicity that surrounds them. The idea of the enema has already been explained. It is certainly impossible to try and deliver a baby easily if the bowel, and particularly the rectum, or back passage, is full of faeces, but not every maternity hospital will feel that an enema is justified if there has been a recent bowel action, especially if there has been an episode of diarrhoea.

2 Rupturing the membranes, or breaking the waters, is another very common procedure and, in fact, is almost always carried out at some point during the induction. If some of the water surrounding the baby is drained off, then the baby's head will go lower into the pelvis. It is the pressure of the baby's head on the neck of the womb that stimulates it to open. Sometimes some of the water behind the baby will be drained off too. The womb, which acts as a sort of pump, works more effectively in pushing the baby down the birth canal if it is not too full up.

3 Finally, a synthetic hormone, in the form of pitocin or syntocinon, may be given to stimulate the womb directly to contract. It may be given as a pill to be dissolved under the tongue, or as a solution directly into a vein by means of a 'drip'. The drip has the advantage of being more easily regulated and more constant in action. But, of course, it does mean a little more discomfort.

I do hope that all these procedures do not sound too terrifying. They are not. In fact they are no more than slightly uncomfortable. If they are all carried out, and they often are, then the doctor will often set up a monitor, or check, on the contractions that are caused and on the baby's reaction to them. This means a wire recording the contractions of the womb and a wire recording your baby's heartbeat. These will be connected to a machine and will give a constant and accurate record of everything that is going on without having to disturb you unnecessarily. None of these is the slightest bit painful.

However, it is not particularly comfortable lying on a hard bed for any length of time and, unfortunately, it remains for some women a rather embarrassing time. You do not need to feel embarrassed. Your midwives and doctors are with you to help you deliver a healthy baby and this must be the aim of everybody. Being in labour cannot be comfortable, but, with proper understanding of what is going on, and with the aid of medicines and the occasional injection to help you, it can be not too painful. And, above all, it is the most rewarding experience that any woman can possibly have. Never be afraid to ask what is going on and rest assured that someone will always be there to help and explain things to you. When the time comes for your baby to be actually born you will find that this is not painful. It is certainly a strange but very wonderful feeling. Understanding something properly will often abolish much of the pain which arises out of anxiety and fear of the unknown.

Normal Labour

Normal labour is divided into three parts:

Stage 1

This is the time when the baby's head is pushing down against the neck of the womb and forcing it to open. This stage is over when the neck of the womb is fully open and clear for the baby to move down into the birth canal. The pains start off very mildly and are very similar to period pains, if you have already experienced those. They become progressively stronger and are often accompanied by a very persistent back pain. Your whole abdomen will tighten up and the feeling will intensify until it reaches a crescendo and then gradually fall away again. You will then have a time of complete rest and then the whole thing will start again. It is absolutely essential that you learn to relax completely between the pains as this gives you time to summon up your energy again and also gives the womb time to rest before its next bit of work. You must learn to breathe deeply, with control, and using your chest muscles. Sometimes clasping your own, or your attendants', hands will focus your mind somewhere other than on your own abdomen. The contractions will get more frequent and will become longer and more effective as you near the end of the first stage. At no time will the doctor allow the pains to become too severe, but he will give you a pain-killing injection, or show you how to breathe using a gas and air machine to relieve the tension which aggravates the pain. However, many women can cope very well on their own once they have mastered the technique of breathing deeply during the contractions and relaxing totally between them. Encourage yourself by knowing that, as the pains get stronger, this means that the womb is working more effectively in pushing the baby down towards the final path to being born. And, also, the stronger the pains are, the shorter will be the first stage, and the nearer you are to reaching the exciting second stage.

Stage 2

This is the stage during which the baby proceeds down the birth canal or vagina to be actually born. It is a very short stage and here your labour can become almost fun. In the first stage all the work is being done by the womb itself and you can do very little to influence it, but when the neck of the womb is finally open, then you can really help. With every contraction of the womb you must take a really enormous breath and push the baby down as hard as you can. This means push as though you have gone to the toilet and are going to have your bowels open. It feels just like that and is very low down and far to the back.

Stages in normal vertex (head-first) delivery

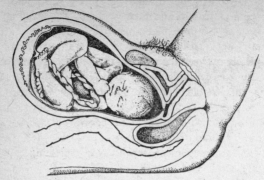

1 Head descends into pelvis

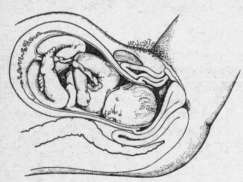

2 cervix opens

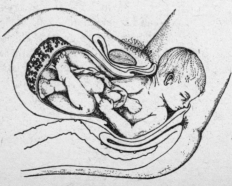

3 Cervix fully dilated. Head appears

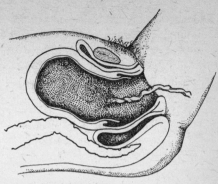

4 Placenta remains

The back passage is right next door to the vagina and the sensation that you feel as the baby comes down is just like that of having your bowels open. When you are actively pushing down like this it does not hurt. You will not feel any pain. It will feel most odd and certainly not particularly comfortable, but it does not actually hurt. One of the commonest worries at this stage is the fear that something is going to split. The vagina itself has tremendous stretching power and no baby is ever too large to pass through. Sometimes the skin at the very outside of the vagina, however, does seem to the doctor to be stretching unduly. If he feels that this is so, he will sometimes make a small cut rather than allow any possibility of a tear, because a cut which is sown up immediately after delivery heals well and easily, whereas a tear can be more difficult.

If the doctor does decide to make a small cut or episiotomy, you may rest assured that you will not feel it at all. He will use a local anaesthetic and you will feel no pain. As the baby's head appears to the doctor or midwife who is with you, you will be told to stop pushing and to pant. This means breathe very fast and very shallowly, in and out. This is to stop you giving that final enormous push which would pop the baby's head out. It is very much safer for the baby to be born slowly at this point. The doctor wants to be able to ease the baby gently out into this

59

world and not have it suddenly pop out which can cause an undue amount of pressure on the very soft skull. Once the baby's head has been born you will be asked to push again and the rest of the baby's body will come. This is comparatively no problem, the head is the largest part of a new-born baby.

Stage 3

The hard part is done. Your baby is born. You will not feel unduly sore, but you will often feel rather shivery and not a little worn out. Unfortunately you have not quite finished. The afterbirth or placenta must be brought out. The doctor or midwife will ask you to give one more small push with the next pain. The delivery of the afterbirth is very easy, although just a little messy.

You will possibly need a few stitches if you have needed a small cut to ease out the baby's head, but this is an undignified procedure rather than an uncomfortable one. You really can relax now and listen to that sound that you had begun to think might never happen; the sound of your baby's first cry. Some mothers are lucky and experience an immediate feeling of tremendous fulfilment. For others this comes later. Do not worry if it is not immediate for you. But do, if you can, take your baby straight to you and, even better, put it straight to the breast. I am convinced that this really does help to cement that very early bond between mother and baby. Let the father have that first new-born cuddle too, especially if you have been fortunate enough to have his help and support during your labour.

Analgesia in Labour

There are many ways nowadays that the pain of labour can be relieved.

1 Early in labour simple pain killing tablets are all that may be required.

2   Later on, the stronger drugs such as pethidine will be given by injection.

3   If your labour is not properly started, then you may well be given something to help you sleep for a few hours so that you may better conserve your energy.

4   Later still in labour, when the pains are very strong, just before the neck of the womb is fully open, your midwife will show you how to use the gas and air machine. By breathing deep and hard into this you help to control your own breathing at the same time as receiving an amount of the pain-relieving gas. This is a marvellous way of acquiring the art of breathing properly, of getting rid of that bit of tension and of taking the edge off the pain at the same time.

5   I have already mentioned the local anaesthetic which is used if you need to have a small cut made right at the opening of the vagina.

6   Recently it has become increasingly common to have a special form of pain-killing injection which is called an 'epidural anaesthetic'. This means that a pain-killing injection is given around the bottom of the spinal cord in the back which stops all pain felt below that level. This means that you cannot feel the contractions of the womb at all, although it has no effect upon the strength or the quality of those contractions. It can, however, mean that because the sensations from your womb or pelvis are absent, you cannot participate and co-operate in your labour so well. Many women learn to overcome this and will push well when instructed to do so by the doctor who can feel the contraction. This does, however, remain an obstacle for those women who wish to participate totally in everything that is going on. However, the vast majority of those mothers who have had their babies in this way have been absolutely thrilled with it and choose this method for preference if they can for their subsequent babies.

Having said all this I must stress that you are by no means obliged to have any analgesiacs in labour. Many women, particularly with a second or subsequent baby, manage perfectly well without analgesia, or with only the very minimum of help. Some people will tell you that with adequate preparation you should be able to abolish the pain of labour entirely. I simply do not believe this to be true. Certainly, as I have already stressed, it is possible to help yourself a great deal by adequate preparation, but I believe that labour remains an extremely individual experience. I have certainly delivered women who experience not only no pain but no discomfort either throughout their labour. But I have also delivered women who have had a complete and very excellent preparation and who, throughout their labour, remain totally relaxed, yet in spite of all this require considerable amounts of analgesia. So I do not believe that you need feel any sense of failure at all if you do require considerable help. There remains a large element of luck in how your individual body reacts and copes with its own special task of having a baby. And those babies are individuals too, so just because you have one rather difficult experience there is no reason to suppose that they would all be difficult.

You owe it to yourself to prepare yourself as well as you are able. But after that has been said some of you will need very little, if any, analgesia, while others will need several injections and the gas and air machine. Whichever is the case, if you achieve the desired end result of a baby, you have succeeded completely.

Variations of the Normal Delivery

1 Forceps delivery is certainly much more common now than it used to be. This is mainly because, in experienced hands, the forceps can facilitate delivery, when either the baby is at risk or the mother getting tired, or if, for any reason, there is a delay in the second stage of labour. I know that many mothers feel 'cheated' if their babies are delivered by forceps apparently at the last minute. But the decision is generally not taken lightly.

It may be that the baby's heartbeat has slowed down slightly, this means that it is having difficulty in the final stages of its birth, and the quicker it is delivered the better. It may be that the baby's head is turned round so that it faces backwards. This is a slightly more awkward way for delivery to take place and it is often safer to apply forceps to turn the head round. It may even be that the mother is getting tired and is not able to push quite so well. Whatever the reason, it will be a good one and one that is taken in the interests of mother, or baby, or often both.

2 In certain circumstances the baby must be delivered by a Caesarian section; that is through an opening made in the abdominal wall, rather than being born in the normal way. This is often a decision that is made before the baby is due, as in the case of a mother with diabetes, a mother whose pelvic measurements are too small, or a mother who has had undue difficulty before. But sometimes it is a decision which must be made instantly because of the condition of mother or baby. It does not happen often this way, but occasionally labour does not proceed smoothly and, if the baby gets distressed and cannot be delivered quickly by the normal route, then it must be delivered by Caesar.

Sometimes the afterbirth is in front of the baby's head and stops the head being pushed down the birth canal. There is nothing for it in these circumstances but to deliver the baby by Caesarian section. Whatever the reason for the operation it does not mean an increased risk to the baby and in some cases may definitely be safer for it. Of course it is not quite as satisfying as delivering your baby yourself but you have done the hard work of carrying the baby for nine months and if it is safer for it to be delivered by operation it is little really to have to give up.

3 Sometimes the baby, instead of being head down in the abdomen, is the other way up. This is a more uncomfortable way of carrying it because the large head pushes up under the ribs. And it is slightly less satisfactory to deliver this way up because the baby's bottom is a less satisfactory opening lever

than the head. For these reasons your doctor will often try to turn the baby from the breech position into the vertex position. This is described in an earlier section of the book. If it is not possible to turn the baby, however, there is absolutely no reason why the baby cannot be delivered quite safely, bottom first. The doctor will often be in attendance at this type of delivery because forceps are usually applied to the aftercoming head to protect it as it is being delivered. An added bonus to this type of delivery is that the baby is born with an unusually beautifully shaped head rather than the slightly elongated version of the vertex delivery!

4   A twin delivery is another that will nearly always be attended by a doctor. There is very little more alarming about a twin delivery than a single delivery. It takes a little longer, because you have to have two second stages rather than just one. And, according to which way up the babies are, it may include a breech delivery as above. You do not have to go through the first stage twice, however, and the second stage of the second baby is very often much easier because the way has already been opened by the first.

What can go Wrong

Things can go wrong in labour, but for the most part they do not. The points listed below are mainly the less serious ones and the most common.

1   Labour uses a lot of energy. This means a constant supply of glucose or some similar energy-giving food must be taken. Similarly, labour makes you very hot and you need to replenish your fluid stores continually. Particularly, therefore, if your labour is a fairly long one, you do need adequate supplies of food and drink. Your doctor will know if you need more fluid, because you will excrete a substance known as acetone in your water. Sometimes it will be necessary to correct this by giving you fluid and glucose via a drip into your arm.

2   In those women who have had toxaemia of pregnancy, it is necessary to watch the blood pressure throughout labour and even for some hours after. Occasionally the blood pressure continues to rise and it is necessary to bring the labour to its conclusion quickly rather than wait for its own natural course. This may mean a forceps delivery or even, very occasionally, a Caesarian section. It may be that to give the mother a general anaesthetic, and deliver the baby, is the safest thing for both, although it can be very galling for the mother who had been progressing well in labour.

3   Occasionally the baby does not come smoothly down the birth canal and may even become temporarily wedged. This will not harm it but, of course, it has to be turned or manoeuvred so that it may continue its journey. Sometimes the doctor will need to turn it with forceps.

4   The placenta or afterbirth is usually delivered very soon after the baby, but occasionally it can get stuck and then it has to be helped out. Once again, very occasionally, this can mean a general anaesthetic. There is always some blood loss when the placenta is delivered and if it gets stuck and has to be removed then there can be extra blood loss. Occasionally the mother will need a small blood transfusion to replace that blood loss.

The aim of the attendant doctor is to achieve a reasonably fast and essentially smooth delivery of a healthy baby and to leave the mother feeling comfortable and fulfilled albeit rather tired. Any occasional departures from the norm will be in order to achieve this end, although I know how frustrating it can be to have the final delivery of your child taken out of your hands when, as far as you know, labour is proceeding smoothly. Nothing pleases the midwives and doctors more than a calm uncomplicated delivery and they will not interfere unless they think that it is in the best interests of mother and baby.

There remain those accidents of birth that cannot be foreseen and cannot often be prevented. They are, very happily, few and far between, although so upsetting and often bewildering to those parents who have experienced them. You will always hear about them simply because of their nature, but I must repeat that they are rare. If something like this does happen to you then I would say, talk to your doctor; talk it out with him until you can come to terms with it. He will often be able to reassure you that the chances of such an accident happening to you again are virtually nil, but in any case he will be able to lay all the facts before you.

The Baby at Birth

Your baby is born and the midwife or doctor will clamp and then cut the umbilical cord. While the baby is actually being born it often gets a bit of mucous in its mouth and this will be sucked out, with the aid of a bit of tube, by the midwife. It is almost impossible not to worry about the strange gurgling sounds that this can produce, but they are entirely normal. The baby will, by this time, be crying lustily and, having been wrapped in a warm towel, will be handed to you for the first and most important cuddle. If you can put it to the breast at this time, it will help the afterbirth to be expelled rapidly and completely.

The average weight of a newborn baby is about $7\frac{1}{2}$lb (3·4kg), but this can vary tremendously. Variations between 6–$9\frac{1}{2}$lb may be regarded as entirely normal. Girls, on the whole, tend to be smaller than boys; children born to tall parents tend to be larger than those born to shorter and smaller parents; babies born before term are generally smaller than those born at or after term; babies born to mothers who have smoked a lot during pregnancy tend to be smaller, and babies born to mothers who have been ill, or had severe toxaemia during their pregnancy, tend to be smaller. There is no particular virtue in having a baby of any particular size, but those babies born at term under 6lb, or thereabouts, will often have a blood test to see if they are short of sugar and need extra feeding, while mothers of babies born over 10lb will require to have a blood test in case they show any tendency to diabetes.

The shape of the normal baby can also vary enormously, particularly the shape of the head. As the baby comes down the birth canal, the head is moulded by the shape of it and the baby can be born with a very elongated head. Breech babies have a characteristically square head. Moulding will resolve and the shape become correct in the first few days of life, but can be quite alarming.

When the baby is first born, the midwife or doctor will award it a score. This is called the Apgar score which is purely a means of assessing how quickly it recovers from the effort of being born. Marks are awarded as to its colour which may range from blue to white or pink; for the pulse which may be fast or slow; for its activity, assessed in terms of the vigour of the cry; for the tone which is a measure of how limp or active the movements are, and, finally, for its breathing which may vary from slow and irregular to fast and strong. Babies vary enormously as to how quickly they recover and this merely gives the doctors and midwives a good guide as to how long they should continue to watch the baby very carefully. For instance, if the baby is pink all over, crying lustily and wriggling all over the cot within a minute of being born, then provided it is warm and nursed on its side in the cot it may be safely left while other things are attended to. But if it is listless and has not got a good cry, then it has probably had a rather more difficult time being born and will need more careful handling and watching for a while. It is easier for the midwives to keep a really close eye on a baby if it is in an incubator and if your baby is nursed in an incubator for the first few days it does not mean there is anything wrong with it but merely that it needs a warm and quiet rest.

After the baby has been delivered and you and your husband have had your first time together with it, it will usually be nursed in the ward nursery for a few hours while you have a well earned period of sleep and recuperation. The baby needs a sleep too, and after a good rest you will both be ready for the first try at feeding.

Much more about your newborn child and how it looks and reacts appears in a later section, but for now I will go on to consider what is really the final stage of your pregnancy—the puerperium or lying-in period. This is the time when the uterus is returning to normal and your hormones are readjusting to feeding, rather than carrying, a baby.

The Puerperium

Medical Aspects of the Lying-in Period

1 Involution is the name given to the shrinking down of the womb to the normal size. This is measured by your midwife feeling the height of the womb through your stomach wall. Usually it will not be possible to feel the womb by the end of the week.

2 As the womb shrinks, so the loss from the vagina will change. At first this will be bright red, becoming pink, and finally brown like the last day of a period, and then it will gradually stop altogether. Some people, however, are unlucky enough to continue with this brown discharge until they have a normal period. The loss stops much more quickly if you are breast-feeding your baby; in fact you may, instead of having a continuous slight loss, only experience loss while you are actually feeding. Although your loss will disappear more quickly if you are breast-feeding, your first period will often be considerably delayed. You may not, in fact, have another period until you have finished feeding. This does not mean, however, that you are infertile during this time and you should take contraceptive precautions. There is more about this in a later chapter.

3 Afterpains are the pains that you feel low in your stomach and which persist after delivery for anything from a single day

to a week. They are really much like sharp and brief labour pains. While you are in hospital you will be offered tablets to relieve these. You may well need nothing, and many women do not experience afterpains at all. But if you do have them, rest assured that they are common and entirely normal.

4 Many women experience some difficulty and soreness when they first try to pass water after delivery. Occasionally this is because it was necessary to pass a tube into the bladder to empty it during the actual birth of the baby. A baby being born needs all the room it can get and a full bladder does interfere with this. It can be very difficult to pass water spontaneously while you are actually in labour and, rather than asking you to keep trying to do something which is not only difficult but also uncomfortable, the attendant will slip a catheter into the bladder for you. If you do experience this difficulty passing water afterwards, do not worry, drink plenty and try to relax and you will, in time, be successful. If any burning on passing water persists, however, it is possible that you have a slight infection and this should be reported.

5 Your bowels also have to recover and it is very important to get these working again promptly. Your midwife will give you something to help if there is any difficulty.

6 Finally, and perhaps most importantly, your breasts will undergo changes. Hopefully you will be planning to breast-feed your baby and during the first few days after delivery they will be filling with milk. This can be a very uncomfortable time, but fortunately it is shortlived. The stimulus to get the milk to flow freely is the sucking of your baby and so the quicker that you can get it to suck well the quicker your breasts will become comfortable. If it is not a very strong sucker, you may have to massage the breasts manually at first. Your midwife will help you with this.

The two things that will help you above all to relieve the tenseness and soreness are: (a) to wear really good support in the form of a feeding bra, and (b) to keep the nipples well lubricated with cream. If you are in hospital you will be provided with cream, and if not your midwife will recommend a suitable brand. Above all, keep the stimulus to the breasts going at regular intervals and do not be tempted to leave one feed out in the mistaken idea that it will ease the breasts. Finally, rest assured that the soreness does not go on long, as, by about the third day, the milk flow will have become properly established and feeding time rather than being something of an ordeal will then become a pleasure.

How Long in Hospital?

You and your doctor will have planned early on in your pregnancy whether you are to be a short-stay, officially forty-eight hours, or a long-stay mother which varies in length from seven to ten days. If you are a first-time mother; have had any difficulty in this pregnancy, or in previous pregnancies; if you have had four pregnancies already; if you have had difficulties in a previous delivery; or if for any other reason your doctor thinks that a slightly longer stay in hospital is advisable, you will be offered the chance to stay in a little longer. If, on the other hand, you had a perfectly uneventful pregnancy before, with a straightforward delivery, you may well elect to stay in for the minimum period of time, to upset the routine of the rest of the family as little as possible. There are so many considerations to be taken into account here and each decision is a very personal one. Have you other children at home? Have you someone whom the children love and trust, and with whom your husband can get on well, who could successfully take over while you are in hospital? Have you the sort of domestic arrangements which would make it possible for you to get adequate rest at home? You and your husband should discuss all this fully before coming to a decision. Of course if you live in an area where the pressure on hospital beds is very great, and you have no medical reasons for staying in a longer time, and your home conditions are reasonable, then it may well be that you are not given the choice. Whatever happens you must remember that you will be tired; you will need adequate rest; your children will tend to be more demanding until they get used to the new arrival; you will not be getting the benefit of an uninterrupted night's sleep while your baby requires a night feed, and I am quite sure that a properly managed lying-in period establishes the smooth running of the household for months ahead. Personally I feel that if you have the opportunity of a few nights in hospital and are happy that your other children and your husband are properly catered for, then you should take advantage of the offer. In spite of the fact that hospitals continue to start the day much too early in the morning, a great deal of the anxiety of those first few days is taken off your shoulders just by knowing that the midwives are always there. This does not mean that you cannot and should not have your baby with you most of the time, but when you are resting, you will, I feel, rest better just by knowing that you are not the only one on duty.

Feelings of Fulfilment

For many of us the time immediately after the baby is born is a very confusing one. You had become used to being pregnant; now you are not. Your body has changed again and in those first few days it is often a remarkably strange and none too beautiful shape! Your baby, which has been quite safely protected inside you, is now independent. It is so often much smaller either than you expected or remembered. It is extraordinarily helpless. Some mothers are lucky and, in spite of this, feel an immediate sense of achievement and fulfilment, even a tremendous sense of togetherness with their newborn child. But by no means is everybody so fortunate. Many of us feel a complete sense of bewilderment at this early stage and it is by no means unusual, even, to feel an element of resentment. Do not worry at this early stage. We have often been conditioned to feel that we will experience an overwhelming sense of love and closeness to our newborn child and many mothers therefore have to

71

endure feelings of guilt if this is not so. These feelings will come and you will not have to force them. Sometimes the feeling that is uppermost in your mind is that of irritation and frustration if, for example, you had to have a forceps delivery at the last minute. This can make you feel very cheated and, instead of a great sense of achievement, you may well feel very let down. This is entirely natural, but try not to indulge the feeling or to feel continuing resentment. Try to wonder at the tremendous fact of birth itself and rest assured that nobody would have taken such a decision if it had not been in the interests of you, your child, or both of you. Finally, those women who have been forced, for one reason or another, to have a Caesarean section, sometimes feel that they have failed in their role of child bearing. It is difficult to reason with this feeling at the emotional time at which it usually occurs, but to me the enormous achievement is the successful carrying of that child for nine months, and if, at the end, it must be delivered by one route and not another, then so be it; you have still successfully born a child, and there can be no greater achievement than this.

Post-natal Depression

This is most conveniently discussed under three main headings. First of all, there is what is commonly termed the 'three-day blues'. This is a period of often acute misery which occurs very soon after the birth of the baby and in which, for most women, the most striking feature is crying—many women are subject to fits of almost uncontrollable weeping. It is generally said that this occurs on the third day, but I have found it at any time from the first day to the seventh. It is a perfectly natural reaction to an enormous physical and emotional strain and is quite logical when viewed objectively. Unfortunately, the hallmark of the condition is that the sufferer is totally illogical and the misery she experiences quite irrational. In fact she very often knows that she is being irrational, but still continues to weep. If you are the sufferer, rest assured that just as suddenly as the depression settled on you, so it will lift. If you are in the position of being comforter to the sufferer, then listen to her, reassure her when you can, and above all tell her that the feeling will go in a very short while. Do not tell her to snap out of it, because she cannot do so.

Secondly, there is the much more insidious, but less acute, form of mild depression brought on by tiredness and the inability to pick up as quickly as you think you should. Much of your figure and energy will pick up very quickly after delivery, but it will be some time before you are completely back to where you were before. This can be most frustrating as you will make tremendous strides in the first few weeks and then things will seem to come to a standstill. You will get back into most of your clothes but not quite into them all. You will love to go out in the evening again but inexplicably you will not have your usual staying power for late nights. If you do not expect this it can make you very depressed. I always explain it in terms of the length of time that you have been pregnant. You have carried your baby for nine months; it is not reasonable in my view to expect to compensate fully for that for another nine months. So try, if you can, to be content to make rather slower progress than you had originally thought. I do not mean that you should be complacent and continue to carry an extra stone around for a full nine months. But, particularly when it comes to waists, wait a little before you throw out your old clothes. You will get back into them. And, finally, remember that nearly every woman who has had a baby experiences this nagging type of depression. In fact one of the very best forms of treatment for it is to talk to someone else who feels exactly the same. You will be amazed at what a tonic that can be!

Thirdly, there is the much rarer, but when it does occur much more serious, true post-natal depression. This does not lift as time goes by, in fact it tends to get worse. It is entirely without reason and cannot be argued against. It can take quite bizarre forms such as increasing absentmindedness and bad memory. It can take the form of a complete inability to cope with everyday chores, or the form of an acute anxiety rather than an actual depression. It is perhaps one of the most difficult things to define clearly. However, if the state of mind of the woman is such that she cannot effectively cope with either the baby or her everyday life, and if the situation seems to be getting worse rather than better, then it is time to seek expert medical help. Sometimes the depression is so acute that there is virtually a crisis and the decision to call for help is not difficult. However this condition can be most insidious and, if the decision to seek the help of a psychiatrist is delayed, it can cause unnecessary suffering. It is a treatable condition and the sooner that it is treated the better for all concerned.

The Midwife at Home

By law in this country, a woman must have midwife care for ten days after her confinement. If you have your baby in hospital, the hospital midwives will look after you during your stay and then your general practitioner's midwife will call daily for the rest of the ten days. She will be able to help you with the day to day care of your baby. She will be able to help you establish a feeding routine. She will check that your womb is going back to the right size satisfactorily. She will be able to help you with all those worries that seem to surround you at this stage. She will be able to allay that panic which so often sets in when you are first on your own at home with your baby. After that ten days you will be able to keep in touch with her through your baby clinic. Do not be afraid to ask her anything. A fear that is expressed is so often a fear halved.

Back to Normal

By the end of ten days, your loss will most often have virtually ceased, especially if you are breast-feeding. Some women, however, do continue to have a slight vaginal loss or spotting until their first period. This should not be red blood, though, and if you have any further red loss you should report it. If you are bottle-feeding, your first period will usually appear anything from four to six weeks after delivery and this period is very often heavier than usual, may last longer, and may even contain a few clots. If you are breast-feeding, however, the first period is often considerably delayed and you may, in fact, not have a period at all until after you have finished breast-feeding. This does not mean that you are infertile during this time and it is possible for you to conceive again even if you have had no period. So it is vital that you do carry out some form of contraception. It is not true that if you are breast-feeding you cannot conceive. The chances of your doing so are diminished, but they are still there.

How soon you resume normal sexual relationships with your husband depends on several factors. If you have had an instrumental delivery, or stitches, you will be sore for a while and it is foolish to try and resume intercourse while this is so. Besides giving no pleasure this might well spoil your enjoyment for longer because you will be tense in anticipation of pain even after it has ceased to become painful. Most women will be reluctant to have intercourse while their loss continues, although this will not necessarily do any harm. But, provided that your perineum has healed, and provided you yourself feel ready for intercourse, there is no reason why you should not get back to normal very quickly. Both you and your husband will often have a very real need of one another at this time. Many women feel that they must wait until their post-natal check at six weeks, but this is not necessary, particularly if your delivery was uncomplicated. Your good sense and the degree of comfort of the perineum will usually be as good a guide as any theoretical timetable. If in doubt, of course, you can always consult your midwife or doctor.

75

It is not wise for so many reasons to become pregnant too soon, so you will need to think fairly quickly about contraception. All methods are open to you after delivery, just as they were before you had the baby.

You do not need to wait for a period before starting the pill, although if you are not breast-feeding, and your period is unlikely to be delayed, then it is perhaps better to wait. If you are breast-feeding, there is a risk, although it is very small, that if you go on the pill your milk supply will dry up. If it is of very great importance to you to feed your baby yourself, it is sensible not to go on the pill for the first few months after delivery. The risk of losing your milk is small, but it is there.

If you would like to have an intra-uterine device fitted the ideal time is at your post-natal examination. You should, if possible, discuss this with your doctor or the hospital before you actually have the baby, although I do understand the natural reluctance of some mothers to discuss contraception before they are delivered.

There is no reason why you should not continue to use a cap and pessary if this was your chosen method before the baby was born. It is possible, though, that you will need a larger cap, at least temporarily, as the tissues of the vagina will have stretched considerably during delivery. Do consult your doctor, your hospital, or the family planning clinic about this, as there is no surer way to reduce the pleasure of renewed intercourse than the fear of another immediate pregnancy. Even if your religion prevents you taking active precautions against pregnancy, do take whatever measures are open to you. The drain on the health of a woman, caused by pregnancies too close together, is very great.

Hopefully your pregnancy has now had a successful outcome and you will now be back into your old pinafore dress even if not your tightest jeans or skirt. Breast-feeding will, with any luck, have become established. If that has not been possible then, hopefully, your baby is settling down into a good routine on the bottle.

In the next section of this book I shall deal with the newborn baby and the immediate problems which it presents.

PART THREE

THE NEWBORN BABY

POUNDS	KILOGRAMS
1	0·5
2	1·0
3	1·4
4	1·8
5	2·3
6	2·7
7	3·2
8	3·6
9	4·1
10	4·5
11	5·0
12	5·5
13	6·0
(1 stone) 14	6·4
(2 stone) 28	12·7

WEIGHT

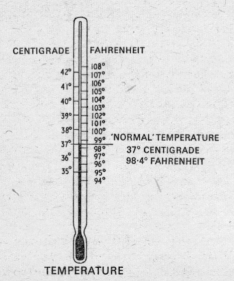

CENTIGRADE   FAHRENHEIT

'NORMAL' TEMPERATURE
37° CENTIGRADE
98·4° FAHRENHEIT

TEMPERATURE

Fig 7   Conversion tables

Getting Ready for the Baby

1 *The Nursery*

Many families will have a separate room for their first baby, although as your family size increases it may be more difficult to organise. In spite of this, I feel happier if a very young baby is sleeping in the same room as his mother. Usually this is not necessary after the first six weeks or so, but a very new baby is really very helpless, and unless you are unlucky enough to have a baby which makes such a noise at night that it stops you getting any sleep at all, then he is safer with you at first.

Soon after the first month, however, you will be able to move your baby into his nursery. Even with subsequent babies, I believe that the first few months of a baby's life are so important in establishing a routine, both for his sake and for yours, that if you can possibly give him a room of his own, it is really worthwhile doing so.

Babies seem to be happier in a light room although the light itself should not be too bright and the cot should not be positioned so that the baby will stare directly at the light.

It is wise to have a room with a window that will open although this must have a safety catch later as your baby becomes a toddler.

The room should be reasonably warm, although it is quite unnecessary to have it too warm. I really do not think it is necessary to have a thermometer in the room; there is great danger in bringing up a baby too much by the book and too little by plain common sense. You can be too scientific about these things. I am very much against a close stuffy atmosphere. I am afraid that the widespread use of central heating and double glazing has predisposed young infants to many more stuffed-up noses.

Apart from any of these considerations, however, probably the most important thing is to make the room functional. Have a flat, safe changing surface with your creams, lotions, powders and cotton wool all readily accessible. Have a rubbish bin within easy reach, and do have a really comfortable feeding chair.

2 *Equipment*

You do not need everything at once. In fact it is a great mistake to get everything at once. Apart from the expense, you will often find that your ideas change as you gain experience and as you watch how other mothers cope with the problems. Also, if you buy things too far in advance, you may well find that they have been considerably improved by the time you actually come to need them. However I really do believe that a carrycot is indispensable. You can, of course, put your baby straight into a cot at night, and use a pram during the day, but a carrycot really does make those first few months simpler. Many people now find the old, large-style pram superfluous and a carrycot with good wheels is all that is necessary. If you can get wheels with a good spring in them, it certainly makes for a much more comfortable ride.

A crib is delightful, but very definitely a luxury. Unfortunately they can be used only for a very short time. You will need a cot soon, even if you have decided not to use one from the beginning. Do check your cot from the safety point of view. It should not have screws that can be easily undone. It should not have balls or other play things that can become easily detached. The bars must be the right distance apart. They should not be so close together that the baby cannot see out clearly and obviously not so far apart that he can get his head out or even partly and thus get stuck. This all sounds very obvious, but I have seen very unsuitable cots on the market. I find that a cot where the mattress can be positioned high or low, is a great back-saver early on. I like the routine of the cot being the place in which your baby will have a long night's sleep and the carrycot being his daytime environment. But I do agree, especially in the case of small babies, that they can get completely 'lost' in a cot in the first few weeks.

These are the only two large items that are necessary in the first few months. It is an added luxury to have a beautifully sprung pram to push along, but so many people now live in flats or up stairs, that it is often impractical to keep a large pram.

3 Bedclothes

Your baby will need sheets and blankets to fit a cot and a carrycot. You will save yourself a lot of bedmaking and your baby a lot of discomfort if you invest in fitted undersheets in each case. All sheeting should be cotton or cotton flannelette from choice. Nylon does not allow the skin to breathe and predisposes your baby to spots especially on the face and neck. There should be a rubber sheet; and I mean rubber and not plastic, underneath the sheet. Again the plastic of most cot mattresses predisposes towards sweat and spots. Babies are much more snug, too, if they have a blanket layer underneath them, particularly in the winter. So I would suggest: a mattress followed by a blanket layer (flannelette will do), followed by a rubber sheet for face and nappy area, followed by a fitted cotton sheet. On top of your baby there will be a sheet (cotton in summer, flannelette in winter) and blankets. These should be safety blankets, cellular, or others specifically recommended for babies. Long-woolled blankets are not safe. You can only tell if your baby is at the right temperature by feeling his forehead and his toes while he is asleep. If both these extremities are warm and dry then he is at the right temperature. If your baby is too hot he will sweat and then he will get spots. He will cry because he is uncomfortable and then his nose will run and then get blocked, and this will further stop him going back to sleep. I have more often seen babies too hot in bed than too cold.

Babies do not need pillows in their first year. Pillows, even baby pillows, are unsafe and should not be used.

4 Clothing

Again I must stress here, do not buy too much too soon, babies grow so quickly. You will certainly need vests, either cotton or wool depending upon what time of year your baby is born. It is not sensible to buy the first size wool vests if your baby is born in June. By the time he is needing them he will certainly be needing a size two if not three. There are people who do not like Babygros, but I do not think that there is any good alternative, especially in the first few months of life. There is certainly no such practical garment. They are warm, they cover all parts of the baby, they are comfortable and are so easily washed. You can always put Angel tops over the top of the Babygro to make your baby look more like a little girl. I would not buy more than three first size Babygros. You will find that you can start using the second size quite early on, unless, of course, your baby is very small at birth.

You will certainly need nappies. I personally use towelling nappies alone and do not use muslin nappies or nappy liners. As you will see from a later section on the subject of nappy rash, I believe that the prevention of nappy rash lies in not leaving a baby in a soiled nappy at all, more than in what type of nappy that is. Probably two dozen nappies will suffice, especially if you are sensible and buy good quality ones. Your nappy pins should be the special safety ones and are best bought in packets of half a dozen. It is amazing how they get lost! You will need plastic pants and, more important than anything else, they should be close enough round the leg to prevent urine leaking out, but they must not be too tight. If they leave a clear mark on the leg, then they are too tight.

There is no doubt that disposable nappies are a tremendous help when you are away or travelling. But they are certainly not as efficient as towelling nappies, and I must say that I have always had to use plastic pants with them if I was not to have all my baby's clothes soiled. They are, of course, also very much more expensive. If changed regularly enough they are probably no more likely to cause a nappy rash that conventional ones, but they do get wetter quicker and therefore need changing more often which, of course, also adds to the cost.

You will probably find that one garment given to you in excess, especially if this is your first baby, is the matinee jacket. So try to encourage your knitting relatives to knit the second or even third size! A woollen bonnet is a necessity for a winter baby, but I must say that I have had very little success with mittens. An all-in-one suit, complete with a hood, would really complete your baby's outfit in style. But, there again, do not get a first size if you have a summer baby.

This is really all you need for the first few months and it is so disappointing not to be able to use all that you are given that it really is worthwhile encouraging your generous friends and relatives to make or buy a larger size. It is probably better to reserve your own buying for later on.

5 *Toys*

Your baby's environment for the first weeks of its life is its cot and pram or carrycot. It will appreciate movement predominantly and then light and bright colour. A gently moving mobile in bright and varied colours is very exciting. Similarly, a string of brightly coloured balls across the cot or pram that it can bang will be of interest. I do not believe that this type of play should ever be unsupervised, however, and do take care that they are the correct distance from the baby. They should be far enough away so that he can just touch them by stretching. Do not put them right in front of his nose.

When choosing rattles do remember that his hand is very small and not strong. So choose a light rattle and one that he can grasp. And do make sure that it has a soft and attractive sound and does not make a harsh strident clatter.

You need no more at this early stage and in fact you can improvise all that I have suggested. You need not buy anything, although of course it is tremendous fun to buy if you are able. A string of wooden spoons and scrubbed cotton reels make interesting playthings.

Your newborn baby, in fact, needs very little play time. He

should sleep for most of the time other than when you are feeding, changing, or bathing him. If you tire him with excessive play he will not have the energy for his next feed and then he will not be able to rest properly after it, and so the vicious circle of a discontented baby will begin.

Finally, I think it is unwise to leave any toys in, or tied to, the cot unattended. This is particularly important at night.

Feeding Your Baby

1 Breast v Artificial Milk

Breast milk is better than any modified form of cows' milk partly because of its constituent parts, and partly because of its added bonus in the form of immunity passed on from the mother. There is no debate about this, so if you can possibly breast-feed your baby, you should. No time is too short for breast-feeding. Any length of time will be of benefit to your baby. Even if you can only manage a few weeks you will have started him off well.

Having said this, however, many other arguments are used both for and against breast-feeding. There will always be somebody to disagree with all of these, but I will point them out, hopefully, to increase the argument in favour of breast-feeding.

1 It is easier. It requires no sterilisation process. It is always 'on tap'. Against this, of course, is the point that there is no deputy. You cannot ask anyone else to give a feed for you. Personally I have always given my babies an occasional bottle feed so that they could be given a feed by someone else in an emergency or if I was delayed for any reason.

2 It is quicker. Again this is simply because there is no washing-up. But of course I would agree that you cannot always breast-feed your baby in company, whereas a bottle seems to be acceptable.

3 It is cheaper. This must be true whatever form of modified cows' milk is used.

4   It is satisfying. There are a few women, but I believe it is only a very few, who do not get a great deal of satisfaction from successfully breast-feeding their child.

I am greatly in favour of breast-feeding, for however short a time, but even if the arguments above carry little weight, there really is no debate as to which is better for your baby. So if you can breast-feed do so.

Having said this, however, there are mothers who dearly want to breast-feed and who, for some reason, cannot do so. Sometimes a premature baby cannot suck and therefore cannot give sufficient stimulation to bring the milk in. Occasionally the nipples crack and although if only one cracks it is often possible to rest it and continue feeding, if both crack you may have to give up. There is no doubt that it is slightly more difficult to establish breast-feeding after a Caesarean section. If either mother or baby is unwell it may be impossible. So if you are not lucky enough to be able to breast-feed your baby, take heart. Very many babies have thrived on the so-called artificial milks and they really are a very good alternative.

2   *Breast-feeding*

Having made the decision to breast-feed do have the courage and perseverance to continue trying until your baby is established on a routine at the breast. Mothers can be put off, particularly at two stages. Right at the very beginning the breasts can be extremely uncomfortable as the milk 'comes in'. And your baby's initial sucks on the very full breasts can be very painful. However, this only lasts a very short while, a few days at the most. Some mothers suffer more than others at this stage and I have found that if the breasts become really full, tremendous relief is gained from just sitting in a hot bath and letting the surplus milk just drip out. It is essential to make sure that the breasts are completely empty after every feed, so when your baby has finished sucking, express the remaining milk if there is any. Good bra support at this stage is important and now is the time to invest in a really good feeding bra. You will, hopefully, prevent sore or cracked nipples by keeping them supple with lanolin or any other recommended cream, in between feeds.

When you have overcome the initial hurdle of the first few days of extreme discomfort, it will all be much easier and your next task is to establish a reasonable feeding routine. There are advocates of a completely random 'on demand' system of feeding, but I cannot support this from either the mother's or the baby's point of view. Certainly your breasts need a feeding routine, or you will find them uncomfortably full if your baby remains asleep longer than usual. On the other hand you will find your breasts unsatisfyingly empty if he demands a feed after only an hour or so. Apart from any other consideration it is impossible for you if there is no time of the day or night when you can reliably bank on being free to do other things.

So I do advocate a reasonably consistent feeding routine. Do not feed your baby at intervals of less than three hours and do not let him go more than five hours during the day. At night, that is between 7 pm and 7 am, if he wishes to sleep for seven or eight hours, there will be few of us who will grumble! But you do need to teach your baby the difference between day and night. The day should consist of fairly regular feeds with fairly regular little play periods. The night should be for sleeping, and if he needs a night feed, this should be given with the minimum amount of fuss and the minimum amount of play. Most of us are, of course, incapable of any other sort of approach in the middle of the night, so tired are we! This may all sound rather harsh for a three month old, but if you do not establish these patterns for your child in the first three months, you will have much greater difficulty in trying to establish them later on.

Of course it all sounds so simple on paper, but in practice it can be absolutely exhausting and intensely frustrating. If your baby wakes and tries to demand a feed after two hours and you are reasonably satisfied that he has had a good feed before, then every minute you spend in trying to trick him into lasting that

88

extra hour will save you hours of frustration later on. If there is a particular time of the day when he is particularly restless between feeds, then choose that time to take him out in the pram. If a baby wakes crying just an hour after a feed, it is very unlikely that he is hungry and almost certain that he is windy. No baby need be picked up the minute that he whimpers, but I would never condone leaving a baby to really cry.

Once you have established a roughly four-hourly feeding routine, your breasts will be perfectly comfortable throughout the day, although when you first start to miss a night feed they will be very full first thing in the morning. This will, of course, mean that the milk will then come very fast and may well make him windy at that first feed. Also you may find that he will take all that he requires in a much shorter time and this in itself can cause him to be frustrated. But, after a few days of the new routine, it all settles down again and it is truly amazing how the breast milk supply will adapt itself to your individual baby's requirements. A lot of the anxiety about breast-feeding is dispelled by understanding these changes and mechanisms.

As your baby grows and takes more feed, you come to the next hurdle in breast-feeding. The times between his feeds lengthen and you may be troubled by an excessive amount of leaking. Many women find that any emotion can precipitate this and some have even found that, by merely thinking about their babies or husbands, they can start a real flow of milk. This can be amusing if you are in the security of your own home but can certainly be embarrassing if you are not. I am afraid that it is sometimes necessary to resort to quite thick breast-pads and often wiser to wear a loose-fitting, patterned dress than a tight, plain-coloured one. Rest assured, however, that if you can overcome this hurdle it will stop and then you will be all set to breast-feed as long as you wish.

I am quite sure that breast-feeding makes you very tired. In some cases, if you have other children already, and perhaps are even trying to continue doing some other work as well, it can make you very tired indeed. I think that this is one very valid reason for not continuing to breast-feed indefinitely. I know that there are some mothers who can continue to seven or eight months quite happily, but I do believe that if you are tired, it is sensible to stop feeding any time after three months. You will certainly not be able to cope with the needs of your baby or the rest of your family if you are permanently exhausted and I am afraid that many of us who are overtired are also bad tempered. If it is your first baby, and your daily routine is not too busy, then by having a short rest before and after feeding and by having a good night's sleep you will remain fit and well. But if you already have children, perhaps even with school commitments, and a busy schedule to your day, I do not think the added energy required to breast-feed for a prolonged period is justified. You have given your baby a good start and it is just as important to him that you remain well and energetic as that you should persevere indefinitely with breast-feeding.

Finally, a few words of caution. Many medicines and drugs, if taken by the mother, will pass into the baby with the milk. Just as in pregnancy, it is unwise to take any medicines or drugs unless specifically prescribed.

If your nipples become cracked and infected, you will need to rest the affected breast and express the milk while doing so. You must seek your doctor's advice about this.

Finally, if you yourself become unwell while breast-feeding, you should ask your doctor's advice as to whether you should continue.

When you are ready to stop breast-feeding, the easiest way to do it is to cut out one feed at a time, thereby gradually increasing the time between each feed that you give. This way if you do it over a period of about a month you will not feel any discomfort at all.

Technique of Breast-feeding

There is a technique to breast-feeding and although many

women, especially if their baby is a good strong sucker, acquire the art naturally, a few points may help those who find it more difficult.

1 The baby finds the nipple by a 'rooting reflex'. If you stroke your baby's cheek gently it will automatically turn towards that stroking finger. So cuddle your baby across your chest and he will turn towards the breast.

2 He cannot suck properly unless he can get hold of an adequate amount of nipple and surrounding breast tissue. It is quite surprising how much breast tissue he will often take into his mouth—often the whole of the coloured area, that is the nipple and the areola. If he only manages to grasp the nipple he is unlikely to be able to suck really effectively.

3 He cannot grasp the nipple properly if it is waving about. So steady it between the thumb and forefinger of the opposite hand so that he can grasp it.

4 He will suck quickly and adequately if he gets a good return for his effort. So massage the breasts gently when he first grasps the nipple to express a few drops of milk into his mouth. He will then 'latch on' much more quickly.

5 You must be relaxed and comfortable when feeding. Sitting bolt upright and tense will not help. So do take time to position both yourself and your baby.

6 The only stimulus to good milk production is the regular and complete emptying of the breast. If at first your baby does not completely empty the breasts at each feed you are well advised to express the remaining milk so that the breasts are adequately emptied every time.

7 The first five minutes of breast-feeding are always the most active, so start your baby off on alternate sides at each feed. Otherwise you will find that you are continually stimulating one breast more than the other. One breast will then be much fuller than the other; you will become lop-sided and your baby will become disinterested in the under-producing side.

8 You should not keep the baby at the breast for indefinite

periods. You will get tired and he will gain very little in any time in excess of ten minutes on each side. So the ideal sort of time schedule is to feed for ten minutes on one side, stop and wind him for five minutes, feed for ten minutes on the other side and, finally, wind him again thoroughly. This gives a total feeding time of half an hour and is quite sufficient.

9 Do not let the baby drop off to sleep while at the breast. You will not have winded him adequately and even if you lay him straight down to sleep, apparently happily, he will wake after an hour or so with wind.

10 Occasionally, in the early weeks, if you are lucky enough to produce large volumes of milk, the milk will come too quickly for a small baby. You can regulate the milk flow by very gently pinching the nipple. But do take care not to pinch it too hard or you will stop it altogether.

Requirements of a Nursing Mother and Failure of Lactation

All sorts of folk remedies are advanced for the increase in breast milk, but there are in fact only four main things that materially affect the supply of breast milk.

1 Adequate diet. All you really have to do is maintain the diet that you had in pregnancy. You must have sufficient calories. You must eat enough of the foods containing the essential vitamins; that is meat, fish, eggs, dairy produce, fresh vegetables and fruit. And, finally, you must take in enough calcium, which means drinking at least one pint of milk in some form or other.

2 You must have an adequate fluid intake. There is no doubt that an increased fluid intake will boost your supply of breast milk, provided that you also have enough rest.

3 Adequate rest. Ideally you should rest before and after each feed, although I realise that this often becomes an impracticability if you have other children. However, you should be able to put aside some part of the day for an added rest and you should be able to manage reasonably long nights.

4 The single best stimulus to good breast-feeding, however,

remains the complete and regular emptying of the breasts and if this is not accomplished by your baby in the early weeks, then you must achieve it by manual expression.

There are people in whom breast-feeding is not a success, and never becomes established. Sometimes this is purely a mechanical problem, the nipples being too small, or inverted. This problem should, however, be possible to foresee and thus to alter while you are waiting for your baby to be born. Sadly, not enough attention is paid to the adequate preparation of the nipples during the antenatal period, so if you are keen to breast-feed, do check with your doctor or midwife to make sure that you do not need nipple shields, or any other form of help. Sometimes the breasts become very engorged and, because it is painful and difficult to feed, they are not properly stimulated and then, of course, the milk supply does not come in.

But probably the commonest reason for not breast-feeding is a combination of anxiety and overtiredness. The anxiety can, in part at least, be overcome by finding out all about it before it is actually time to start. With any luck you will be able to get to know someone who is feeding successfully and to appreciate their obvious satisfaction and enjoyment. Your midwife will be able to answer a lot of your questions and many are extremely helpful when the time arrives. Many people are worried that they never know the amount the baby is actually taking, but this is really a temporary problem only and of course you can always test weigh your baby.

You will never successfully breast-feed if you are always over-tired and you must be prepared to take life that bit easier for as long as you do feed. The satisfaction of feeding is certainly great enough to merit time and patience in the first few weeks and I do most strongly recommend it.

I know that for some people there is absolutely no appeal in the thought of breast-feeding and, in fact, for some the idea is almost abhorrent. I can appreciate this view, but even among this group I am sure there are those whose dislike is rooted in fear and anxiety. The only possible hope is, again, to get to know and understand someone who is deriving great pleasure from it. But if, after doing this, in all honesty, you still dislike the idea of breast-feeding, then it is not worth pursuing. You will get no satisfaction and neither will your baby if you are permanently tensed up.

3 Artificial Feeding

Of course there is nothing artificial about the alternatives to mother's milk that are on the market. They are all cows' milk modified in some way or other so as to preserve them. They are then reconstituted in various ways so that as near as possible they resemble mother's milk. You can start off with fresh milk, powdered milk, or evaporated milk. These have to be treated in different ways so that they more nearly approximate human milk.

Powdered milks which have the advantage of having vitamins (except vitamin C) already added, are mixed in a sterile way with boiled water and added sugar. There are a number of powdered milks always on the market and there is very little difference between them. There are one or two with extra additives for use with babies with a particular problem and on these your clinic or doctor will advise you specifically. All the others are fairly standard provided they are made up exactly according to the instructions. The only really important rule about making up any of the powdered milk preparations is to make absolutely sure that you do not overfill the measuring spoon and that the milk thereby becomes more concentrated. I have seen many examples of the mother who thinks to give her baby an added boost she will just pop in another half measure. She then makes the bottle up to the original or usual volume. This can be extremely dangerous, as the baby will not be able to cope with the increased strength. You must stick to the measures and volumes on the instructions of whatever milk you choose to use.

If you try one of these powdered milks and your baby thrives, there is no need to look any further. Stick to that choice. If you are recommended a particular milk then I would go along with that recommendation. If your baby seems unhappy, is excessively windy or tends to regurgitate rather a lot at every feed, then by all means try a change of milk. If this does not help him ask your doctor's advice. Do not keep on chopping and changing, you will only make the situation much worse. I have seen more babies consistently regurgitating through faulty technique than through the wrong milk. And sometimes, I am afraid, there are babies who always will bring up a little of every feed, whatever you do. Provided the baby thrives and continues to put on weight, there is no cause for alarm.

Evaporated milks are diluted with boiled water and then sugar is added in a similar way. The instructions for quantities are fully given on the side of the tin. The advantage of evaporated milk is that it does not go into lumps on mixing. But it has no additives and you must give extra vitamins and separate, extra, vitamin C.

I would not recommend fresh milk under three months, and when you do change to it, it should be made up with 1oz of water (boiled) to the amount of feed given. For instance, if your baby takes a 6oz feed, he will have 5oz of boiled fresh milk with 1oz of boiled water and $\frac{1}{2}$–1 level teaspoonful of sugar added. As the baby takes a larger feed, so the concentration of feed taken will increase. When he has been taking an 8oz bottle for a month (that is 7oz of boiled fresh milk and 1oz of boiled water), you may stop adding the boiled water. After this it is wise to gradually decrease the amount of added sugar. Fresh milk should be supplemented with vitamins.

Technique of Bottle-feeding

1   Most babies do best on a medium-size holed teat. A large hole in the teat will mean the baby gets the feed too quickly and he will almost certainly get a stomach ache. The time taken for the complete feed should not be less than fifteen minutes. He

will not be satisfied if he does not have adequate sucking time. He will then cry because he wants to suck for longer, but he will be full up and so any further feed will only give him indigestion.

2   A hole that is too small will mean that he has to work too hard for too small a reward. He will get tired and fall asleep underfed. He will then wake early and demand more.

3   Cold feeds do sometimes seem to cause colic, although there are babies who tolerate them well. As a general rule you should rewarm the bottle by standing it in a basin of warm water while you are winding the baby, half-way through the feed.

4   You will need to teach the baby to let air into the bottle, although most babies seem to learn very well by themselves, or even in spite of us! Encourage him to release the teat periodically, by turning the bottle in his mouth or even removing it to let the air in. But do not keep on removing the teat, or you will really make him cross. Later on he will do the releasing by himself.

4   Additives

1   All babies require vitamin supplements whatever type of milk they are being fed on. Your clinic will provide you with a standard vitamin preparation which will certainly contain vitamins B complex and vitamin D. For most milks, vitamin A is present in sufficient quantity. The exact amount of vitamin preparation which is required with each type of milk is usually shown on the instruction leaflet supplied with the vitamin drops. Vitamins should continue to be given until your baby is on a complete mixed diet.

2   There are vitamin preparations which contain vitamin C as well but it is wise to give this particular vitamin in the form of a separate drink such as Delrosa or Ribena. This is a wise addition to your baby's diet even when he has started mixed feeding.

3   Probably all babies would benefit from the addition of a small amount of iron to their diet and many of the powdered

milks do incorporate this already as do some vitamin preparations.

It is impossible to be more specific than this as practices do vary. So be guided by your particular clinic. But, as a general rule, you should give the recommended vitamin preparation in the quantity appropriate for the type of milk you are using. You should give added vitamin C in the form of a vitamin C concentrated fruit drink and this should start by the end of the first month. A full-term, normal sized baby will not require anything else, but a premature or small baby might well be recommended specific iron drops in addition.

5 Volumes of Feed Required

Your baby requires $2\frac{1}{2}$oz of prepared milk per pound of his body weight each twenty-four hours (150ml per kg). A quick way to calculate this in pounds is to say that he requires half his weight as pounds in ounces, five times per day.

Hence a 10lb baby requires:

$$10 \times 2\frac{1}{2} = 25\text{oz per day}$$
$$\text{or } 10 \div 2 = 5\text{oz 5 times per day}$$

The total volume of milk feed required in twenty-four hours may be easily read from the graph on p 102. Simply divide the volume required by the number of feeds to be given in one day. You will not do your baby any harm by varying these amounts slightly but this guide will ensure his steady growth without his getting fat.

If you are breast-feeding, the volume of milk taken at different times of the day varies enormously, particularly if you have periods of intense activity yourself during the day. So if you decide to find out how much your baby is taking from the breast by test-weighing him (see below), it is no good at all weighing at only one feed. All the feeds in a twenty-four period must be tested. Your bottle-fed baby will also show a variation in his requirements from feed to feed, but to nowhere near the same extent.

97

Your baby will require very little in the way of other fluid in the first month, but it does no harm to offer a little boiled water in the afternoon, especially if the baby is restless. From the first month onwards, you should offer him a vitamin C fruit drink once a day. It is obviously wise to offer this during the period of the day that the baby is most restless. Certainly do not wake him in order to give it.

During hot weather your baby may well require considerable quantities of fluid other than milk. It is no use trying to ease his thirst by further milk feeds; you will only make him fat and leave him still thirsty. Certainly the summers of the last few years have made this a real problem for babies born in the height of this season.

Complementary and Supplementary Feeding

These are the terms used for topping up your baby if he appears still hungry after a breast-feed, and for the system of giving a bottle feed in between breast-feeds, supposedly to allow the breast to fill better. I think that both these practices are fraught with danger unless they are done for a very short time and are really properly supervised by someone who knows what she is doing. I have already explained that the greatest stimulus to breast-feeding is the regular and complete emptying of the breasts. Therefore if you only feed three times in the day instead of five, the breasts will, in a very short time, learn to fill only three times in the day. There are very short term problems that can be managed in this way, but they are very few and far between.

There is a greater case to be made out for the supplementing of a breast-feed in the early days when your own milk supply has not become properly established but this should only be necessary for a very short while. Do get your midwife's help in this and, if necessary, test-weigh your baby regularly to see how far short of his requirements your own supply is. There is nothing more exhausting and frustrating than having to give a breast-feed and a bottle-feed every time, and if this becomes a pattern I'm afraid it is sometimes worthwhile changing over to a bottle completely. There are mothers, however, perhaps who are working part time, who find that at one feed during the day they have little milk but at all other times are feeding well. If this is the case, then I am sure it is worth continuing with the breast-feeding, because your baby will derive such benefit from it.

7 *Other Food in the First Three Months*

Almost without exception there is no need for solid food of any sort during this period. In fact it is dangerous to give solid foods too early. A baby does not require solid food until it is dissatisfied with an 8oz milk feed. As you will see by the calculation above, you will not be making up an 8oz feed for him until he weighs about 15lb and the average baby will not be approaching that until he is nearly three months old. The only exception to this rule, then, must be the baby who is very large at birth and whose weight gain is such that he requires an 8oz bottle before he is three months old. This is a generalisation, as all discussions on feeding and weight must be, and there will be babies who do require additional solid food before they are three months old. Similarly, there will be babies who are more content on some solid food before they weigh 15lb. But, nevertheless, general rules are invaluable as a guide line, and certainly it is positively harmful to give a baby solid food too early.

Another thing that is so often done wrongly is to give too large a quantity when the solid food is introduced for the first time. When you first give solid food, give a single teaspoonful. This represents quite a large addition to your baby's diet. It is all too easy to give your baby indigestion in these early stages.

The question of weaning and the types and quantities of food to be tried is fully discussed in the next part of this book.

8 Test-Weighing

This is applicable, of course, only to those mothers who are breast-feeding. If your baby is mostly cheerful and sleeps for good long periods, the chances are that he is getting plenty to eat. But if he seems a rather fretful and discontented baby, then the question always arises as to whether he is getting enough food. The only way to find out is to test-weigh him. As I have explained already, the different feeds of the day are likely to vary quite dramatically in amount, therefore any test-weighing should not be carried out on an isolated feed, but on every feed during twenty-four hours.

This is a time consuming process and I do not believe it should be done lightly or all that often. It often seems to make the mother unduly anxious at feeding time rather than serving to allay her fears. However, if there is serious doubt as to whether the baby is getting enough feed, there is no other way to find out and at least you can give a definite answer one way or another.

In order to test-weigh your baby you must weigh him before and after his feed without changing his clothes or his nappy in between. The difference between these figures will be the amount of feed taken. It is, of course, most important to leave the clothes and the nappy unchanged because the weight of a large motion could completely invalidate the test. If your baby weighs 10lb before a feed and 10lb 5oz after it, then he will have taken 5oz of milk from you. If you add up the total taken in twenty-four hours and then check with the calculation above, you will have a fair idea of whether your baby is getting an adequate feed. It is far more valuable to test-weigh every feed for twenty-four hours than to test an isolated feed every day.

9 Weight Gain

There can be few subjects which occupy as much of the early discussion of your baby than his weight gain. His weight gain has become, in many minds, synonymous with general progress. I do think that it is a great mistake to lay down rigorous laws as to how much your baby should or should not gain and it is far more important that he gains regularly and is a happy contented baby than that he is gaining more or less than your friend's baby. The average weight gain of a child in the first three months varies from 4–8oz per week. Having said that, of course, there are babies who regularly put on only 3oz per week and who thrive. But I am definitely usually happier with a baby who keeps within these bounds, than one who gains considerably more. Even having said that, however, there are babies who, in spite of being purely breast-fed, gain up to 1lb a week initially. Often the period of this intense growth slows down after the first few weeks. So here are some general guidelines which I think are of far more value than any didactic table of expected weight gain.

1 Your baby should be content.

2 His weight gain should be regular from week to week.

3 Usually his weight increase will be more than 3oz but less than 9oz.

4 He will roughly double his birth weight by the time he is five to six months old.

A percentile chart is the type of weight chart normally used by child health doctors. A child whose weight falls on the fiftieth percentile will have half of the children of the same age and height heavier and half of them lighter than he is. He is therefore truly average. There are similar percentile charts for height, according to age and sex. The important thing about such charts is not on which percentile your child falls, but on whether he continues on the same percentile as he grows.

I have resisted the temptation to give an average weight gain chart, for it seems to me that these alarm more often than they reassure. Some mothers tend to watch the chart more closely than they watch their child. It is important for your child to gain steadily according to the guide lines given above. It is of

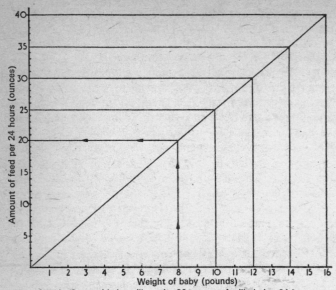

e.g. An 8 pound baby will require 20 ounces of milk during 24 hours
This could be given as 5 feeds of 4 ounces each.

Fig 8   Calculation of amount of feed needed

no value to your child for him to put on weight faster than all
the other children in your area. If he does, the chances are that
you are overfeeding him and he will just become too fat. Many
observers will say that the eating habits of a lifetime are laid
down in the first three months. I believe this to be a slight
exaggeration, but I certainly do think that fat babies often become fat adults. And I know from my own observations that
babies who are grossly overweight in the first six months of life,
show evidence of the failure of the kidney to cope with the extra
food. Mostly, I admit that overfed babies will have been weaned
far too early and often weaned on very unsuitable food. So
stick to milk correctly made up while your baby is content on
milk alone, and when you are ready to start some solid food,

do make sure that you give small quantities of the right sort of foods.

10 *Technique of Winding*

Whichever way you are feeding your baby, whether by breast or bottle, you will need to wind, or burp, him. Time taken at feed time to wind him adequately will save many a frustrating wakeful period. Your baby should sleep for about three hours or so after an adequate feed, and needs to sleep that much. If he wakes after just an hour, it is almost certainly because he has colic from not bringing up his wind adequately at the feed before. This is not always your fault! Some babies are extremely bad at bringing up their wind and you may have to resort to the most extraordinary tricks to help them do so. Some babies are very greedy and greatly resent being taken from the breast or bottle just as they are enjoying a good feed, but you must always wind him half-way through. I have often resorted to putting my baby over my shoulder and walking round the house patting his back in order to divert him long enough to allow him to bring up his wind. Sometimes a very satisfactory burp emerges after only a few minutes, but it can take up to ten minutes. Longer than that is probably a waste of time. If there is still no burp, give a little more feed and try again.

There is often controversy as to whether to change a baby before or after a feed. The 'gastro-colic reflex' that makes a baby open his bowels while he is feeding often makes changing him before a feed a waste of time. So, generally speaking, I think it more sensible to change afterwards, but do remember that he has a very full stomach and do not disturb him unduly while you are changing him.

Babies should be laid down after their feeds either on their sides or on their stomachs so that any surplus wind or milk can be safely brought up. If they do not like being flat on their stomachs and many do not, you can keep them on their sides by rolling up a blanket behind their backs.

103

Personally I have always found it very much easier to feed a baby when it is cosily and well wrapped up. I am sure that four flailing limbs do impede the ease with which you can feed him.

11 *The Crying Baby and the Importance of Routine*

For some reason, perhaps, your baby is not the picture of contentment that you had hoped for.

First of all you must remember that the only way a baby has of communicating is by crying. We often take the fact of his crying as a reflection on our ability to satisfy him when it may simply be a method of communication. So answer the call on the assumption that it is a matter that can be readily dealt with and not as yet another challenge held out to you by your opponent, your baby. A baby does have different cries for different problems and it will take you a little time to learn these. So all you can do in the initial few weeks is try and put right all the usual reasons for crying. When you are satisfied that you have seen to them all, then put the baby firmly down in his carrycot and close the door behind you. I do not mean that you should leave him to scream for hours, but a baby will often whimper or moan slightly for a while before going off to sleep and you must allow him to do that. You cannot expect him to go down without a murmur every time. He will very quickly learn that he is going to be picked up if you always run to him the moment that he wakes or murmurs. So make a determined effort to go away and do some other job for at least ten minutes and then creep back and look at him. He will usually have gone peacefully to sleep by then. But if he is still fretful then do check that:

1   He has not got more wind to bring up.

2   He is in a comfortable position in bed and not lying on his hand or arm.

3   He is clean and dry.

4   He is not just thirsty (I mean for water and not for further feed). This is particularly important for babies born during very hot weather.

5 If he did not finish his feed he does not want it now. Sometimes that wind you have been struggling to get up for ten minutes comes up with ease the moment you lay him down in bed, and this, of course, leaves a gap in his stomach which, justifiably enough, he wishes to be filled!

6 He is warm.

7 He has not brought up a small amount of excess feed and is having to lie in it.

Having said all this and having checked everything, there will still be occasions when your baby remains fretful. Most babies have a wakeful period during the day and you are lucky if it is during the morning or afternoon and not during the evening or night. If he is fretful during the daylight hours then make this the time that you go out, either walking with the pram, shopping or visiting. Somehow a wakeful baby is never so alarming if you are sitting having a cup of tea with a friend. It may in fact even be enjoyable—the friend may even take over the nursing for a while! If you have other children already you will find that the ideal routine is simply not practical, particularly if you have to take or fetch them to and from school. But, whatever your commitments, do try to have some kind of routine in your day. A baby thrives on routine and if he is constantly rushed and bundled here, there and everywhere, then, I am afraid, he is bound to be fretful. You will find that you can disorganise him for a morning or an afternoon, but not for both. And whatever else you do, try and make bathtime, last feed time and bedtime a ritual. That way he will learn that going to bed happens in a certain way at a certain time and he will respond to it. That is, of course, if you value your evenings and your own night's rest as much as I do! You can cope with virtually anything during the day, provided that evenings and nights are peaceful. So aim, above all, to establish the bedtime routine and your life will be so much easier.

Of course this blissful state of affairs will not be achieved in the first few weeks. Most babies of average weight require a night feed for at least six weeks or so and some for longer. However, usually by about six weeks, they will drop one feed, and hopefully this will be the 2am one. Sometimes, however, a baby will drop the 10pm one first. This can be extremely irritating and it is worthwhile waking him at about 11pm for a late night feed and then hoping he will go through to the early morning feed. I am afraid, however, that this does not always work and then the only thing that you can do is to try and prolong the time of uninterrupted sleep and perhaps go to bed earlier yourself so that you, too, get an adequate rest period. It is an odd thing, but babies often seem to drop a feed suddenly and completely just when you are thinking that you simply cannot get up any more at two or three in the morning. In fact it is worthwhile trying to trick him if he seems to go on demanding a feed for too long, by lifting and changing him and just resettling him.

All these generalisations about the management of feeding times and the dropping of the night feeds must remain generalisations. All babies are individuals and must be treated as such. And most mothers who have had several babies will agree that each of their babies had to be treated in a slightly different way. So play it by ear. But I do think that it is worth treating the night feeds simply as feeds and not encouraging the baby to have play periods during the hours of darkness. I have always chatted and played with my children during the daytime feeds but carefully avoided doing so, or overexciting them during the night feeds.

Time given to establishment of a routine at this early stage can save hours of time and frustration later on. I do believe that these first few months are so important for you and your baby. So do try to be firm and fair.

12 Sterilisation Techniques

If you are breast-feeding your baby all that is required is attention to your personal hygiene, a daily bath if that is possible and cleaning of the nipple and the surrounding area just before feeding.

If you are bottle-feeding, however, you will need to adopt some adequate method of sterilising your equipment and of making up your feeds in a clean way. Bottles may be sterilised by using one of the hypochlorous solutions that are on the market, eg Milton. If you use these you must follow the instructions on the packet or bottle carefully. Alternatively, glass bottles may be boiled for three minutes in a large saucepan. Do not forget, if you do use the boiling method, that the bottles themselves must be filled with cold water and submersed before boiling begins. With all sterilisation procedures, cleaning the teats is the most important thing. They should be rinsed really thoroughly under running water to remove all traces of milk and then sterilised by whatever method you have decided upon. I think that it is wise to keep the utensils, jugs, spoons and saucepans, as well as bottles and teats, for the baby only and not to use them for anything else.

Personally I feel that it is better to make up one feed at a time and I know that many people will hold up their hands in horror at this. But I can honestly say that I have not found that it takes any longer to do this and at least you have the comfort of knowing that the feed is fresh and cannot have been contaminated. Obviously if you are travelling or going out, then it is sensible to make up a feed and take it with you, but you should not try to keep it warm until you need it. You should allow it to cool naturally in a closed sterile container and then reheat the feed by standing the bottle in a container of very hot water.

Routine Baby Care

1 Skin and Bathing the Baby

A baby's skin is very soft and delicate and there is nothing quite so satisfying as to see it glow with health, therefore it is important to try and avoid the rashes and spots that so often beset the newborn baby. One of the commonest of these is the sweat rash which is found, in particular, round the face and neck. I have dealt with this a little before in the section on bed-clothes, but it is information well worth repeating. There is no doubt that nylon in clothing and bedding predisposes towards sweat rash. There are babies, of course, who can wear nylon with no trouble, but if you have any trouble at all, do change to cotton clothing, particularly underwear, and cotton sheets. If you have a baby who tends to dribble, cut up one sheet and use it to renew the baby's sheet directly under his face. Matinee jackets and dresses that have fussy ties around the neck are best avoided. Babies do not have a real neck at this early stage and these clothes just tend to rub. A rubber sheet under the cot sheet will protect the baby from the plastic which covers most cot mattresses. I must say also that I have more often found babies to be overdressed than underdressed. It is true that a very young baby needs more clothing than an adult, but be guided by what you are wearing yourself. If you are only wearing a light summer dress then there is no need for your baby to be wearing a vest, Babygro and matinee jacket.

A daily bath is a good thing to establish fairly early on, mostly because the baby's bottom needs to be properly bathed once a day while he is untrained. But there is no need to be completely dogmatic about this, especially in the first few weeks, provided that you cleanse the bottom adequately some other way, for example with a good baby lotion. Your baby will often not enjoy his bath for the first few weeks—it is a strange experience, just like so much that he has to learn. But he will get to enjoy it and will do so very much quicker if you make sure that he does not become frightened at any stage. When bathing him, use shallow water and always keep a supporting hand behind his head so that he can see you at all times. It is not vital to have a special baby bath but a baby will often be less frightened, and become cold less quickly, in a smaller bath. I have always used a hand basin or even the sink in the early weeks. Later, provided that your bathroom is reasonably warm, you can very quickly graduate to a little water in the ordinary bath. This does have its advantages if you have older children too. The baby can have a few inches of bathwater first, and then a toddler or older child can jump in and have some more water. Nearly all children enjoy a communal bathtime and it becomes easier to establish your routine later on. Never leave your baby unattended in the bath; a few minutes are all that he requires and he should then be lifted out and cuddled in a towel, preferably warmed.

There are all sorts of baby soaps on the market and these, in the early weeks, are kinder than ordinary soaps. I have always used Infacare in the bath in preference to a soap at all, mainly because if it does go into your baby's eyes it will not sting. Also it makes a useful baby shampoo which is gentle for a very soft scalp. Babies do like a warm bath although they cannot tolerate the same temperatures as adults. But, in an effort to avoid burning your baby, do not give him a cold bath. He will certainly cry then and very quickly learn to dread bathtime. And do remember that a shallow bath gets cold much quicker than a deep one.

The timing of your baby's bath does not really matter, but a bath is quite a tiring thing for a newborn baby and he will usually sleep very well after it. Also, if you have a toddler already, it is much easier to have one bathtime than two. I can see little value in establishing a morning bathtime only to change it, at six or nine months, to an evening one.

2 Nappies and Nappy Washing

There are several ways of putting nappies on and different authorities will have very different views as to which is the best method to adopt. The best one is the one that you find the easiest and the one that the baby finds the most comfortable

109

leaving his legs free to move. The nappy must not be tight around the baby's abdomen or legs, and remember that the size of his stomach varies enormously with the feed that he has just had. Remember also that if you want to keep the rest of his clothes dry, you must make sure that the whole of the nappy is contained within the plastic pants he is wearing. If a part of the nappy is coming out below the plastic pants then the urine will leak down and soil the rest of his clothes. This can become very expensive and time consuming in washing.

I find the kite method the neatest, and the method most readily adapted to the size and shape of the baby. This and the other common methods are illustrated.

It is generally unwise to use strong detergent or biological washing powders on your baby's clothes. It is probably wisest to start off with a pure soap powder, such as Lux, in the early days and then go on to the milder soap powders, such as Fairy Snow. It is wisest to avoid the biological washing powders altogether.

You must establish a good nappy-washing routine early on. The easiest way to do this is to have a bucket filled with a nappy-cleaning solution, such as Napisan, into which you can just drop the wet nappies. Soiled nappies must be rinsed off first, and I always do this straight down the toilet. When the bucket is full, usually after about six or eight nappies, empty it and wring the nappies out and then just wash them with the rest of the baby clothes. With some of the nappy-cleansing solutions, the manufacturers claim that no further washing is necessary. If you do not use any further washing routine you must be sure that the nappies are rinsed completely free of the solution. There is no surer way of irritating your baby's tender skin and making him prone to nappy rash than to leave some of this strong solution to come into contact with his skin.

3 Prevention of Nappy Rash

A daily bath will go a long way to preventing that most com-

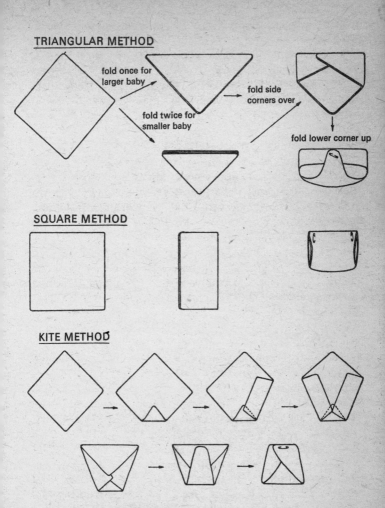

Fig 9   Methods of folding nappies

mon of problems, nappy rash. The other principles to observe though are:

1   Never leave your baby's bottom wet or dirty for longer than is absolutely necessary.

2   Protect the skin on which he lies with a good sticky cream and do remember that if your baby lies on his front to go to sleep it is the front that needs protecting more than the buttocks themselves.

3   Cleanse the buttocks gently but adequately.

This does not mean wake the baby every hour in order to change his nappy. Nor does it mean scrub him at every change. But if you know that he has just passed a motion then change him. And if his bottom is very dirty, liberal quantities of lotion, ie Johnson's Baby Lotion, will cleanse him thoroughly and yet smoothly. There is no better barrier cream than ordinary vaseline if your baby has a tendency to nappy rash, although any of the recommended baby creams is suitable for daily use. There is no greater virtue in one that costs more, and zinc and castor oil cream continues to be perfectly adequate. It really is not worth *not* cleansing the nappy area properly at every change. You will find it infinitely harder to clear up a nappy rash than to prevent one.

There will be times, however, when your baby will be definitely more prone to nappy rash than at others. If he has diarrhoea, or if he is teething, the very nature of his motion makes it more irritating and therefore more likely to make him sore. The treatment of nappy rash is dealt with in a later section.

4   Hair and Scalp

The skin of your baby's scalp is just as tender as the rest of him and it also has soft places, or fontanelles, where the skull bones remain open for some time after birth. So do be careful when washing or attending to the head, but do not forget that it does need regular washing. Even if your baby has very little hair, or none at all, he should have a scalp wash. This does not need to be every day, however, and two or three times per week is perfectly adequate. Again, I use Infacare because it does not sting the eyes if you do inadvertently touch them, and because it is very gentle. The adult anti-dandruff shampoos are too strong for a baby's head and should not be used. It is best to stick to a specific baby shampoo.

Many babies form oily scales or cradle cap on the top of their heads in the first few months of life. This can be very unsightly. It is comparatively easy to remove when mild but extremely difficult to remove if allowed to remain and become very thick. In its mild form, daily use of a gentle baby shampoo, with firm massage to the scalp, will remove the scales. Do not scratch the scalp with your finger nails because this will only aggravate the situation. But there is no reason why you should not massage the scalp very firmly, provided that you use the balls of your fingers. Do not, of course, press hard over the fontanelles. If the cradle cap persists in spite of this regular treatment, then you should see your doctor who will prescribe something stronger. As with nappy rash, this is another of those things that is so much easier to prevent than to cure, particularly once it has got a hold. Cure, then, can be long and tedious.

5 *The Umbilical Cord*

When your baby is first born, the umbilical cord, through which he has been fed while in the womb, is clamped close, so that bleeding cannot occur. Practice varies as to whether this is a plastic clamp, elastic band, or simply a piece of string. But, however it is done, it is clamped a short distance from the skin itself which leaves anything from $\frac{1}{2}$–$1\frac{1}{2}$in of cord to dry up. This gradually shrivels up to become a rather unpleasant-looking blackish stump. This and the surrounding skin, should be cleansed with spirit every day, preferably dusted with an antiseptic powder, such as Sterzac, and then covered with a clean, dry dressing of gauze. Sticking plaster is unnecessary and the stump is much better left open to the air to dry. Try to secure your nappy so that it does not cover the healing cord. If you make sure that every part of the nappy is contained within the plastic pants, you will find that the cord stump, and incidentally all the rest of the clothes, remains clean and dry. After a variable interval, from about four to ten days, the cord will separate and leave a clean stump. Do not fiddle with the cord stump. Do not try to pull it or ease it off. It will separate in its own good time. You only cause it to become infected if you interfere. If at any time it appears red or inflamed and, particularly, if there is any sign at all of inflammation of the skin, you should report it immediately to your doctor or midwife.

6 *The Baby's Motions*

When your baby first passes a motion, it will be dark green, sticky and extremely difficult to clear up. This particular type of motion is called meconium and will last from twenty-four–forty-eight hours. If you have your baby at home during this time, I would strongly advise you to use disposable nappies. It is extremely difficult to launder a nappy filled with meconium. After this, the motion will gradually change to the normal colour and consistency. The transition stage is called the changing stool and is greenish brown, but not nearly so sticky. Finally the motion will settle down to a soft yellow one. If your baby is breast-fed, the stool is characteristically like soft mustard and does not smell. If your baby is bottle-fed the stool is still yellow, but harder, and it does have a smell.

In the early weeks a baby will often pass a motion with every feed, but this will soon settle down. Bottle-fed babies generally have just one or two motions a day, but breast-fed babies can vary very greatly in the number of stools that they have. They may continue to have one with every feed or they may have them much less often, even every two or three days. It does not matter what the pattern is so long as it is reasonably consistent.

The abnormal motion is one that varies from your baby's

114

established pattern, or one that changes colour. There should not be any blood in the motion. If the motion becomes copious and green and contains little solid matter, then the chances are that your baby has an infection. You should report this to your doctor promptly. If, however, the stool becomes very small and green then it is possible that your baby is being underfed. It can be very dangerous to draw the wrong conclusion from the appearance of your baby's motions and you should consult your doctor if you are worried. And remember that if you can show your doctor what the motion is like it is infinitely more helpful than any amount of description.

7 Care of the Eyes

Babies are very prone to getting sticky eyes. Regular daily cleansing with cotton wool dipped in warm water will help to prevent this. But if a sticky discharge or crusting on waking should persist, then you should seek help.

8 Cleaning the Nose and Ears

A newborn baby cannot breathe through its mouth and it is important therefore to keep the nostrils clear. Cotton buds are very useful here but it is just as effective to screw up the corner of a tissue and to rotate it in each nostril. This method does have the advantage, too, of being safer. You cannot push the soft end of a piece of tissue too far or too hard in the nose or ears, but it is possible to do damage with the harder end of a cotton wool bud.

Ears should be cleaned regularly too, and here I do think that the corner of a bath towel or again the corner of a tissue is preferable. It is comparatively easy to damage an ear drum with a cotton bud which is really too rigid. Whatever you choose should be dry, or at least the final clean should be dry. Moisture left in the ear causes the wax, which is a normal secretion, to swell and become a greater problem. Any discharge from the ear is abnormal and should be reported to your doctor. It is alarming how many problems with hearing in later childhood may be attributed to an undiagnosed and untreated infection of the middle ear in infancy.

9 Care of the Mouth

If your teats and feeding utensils are properly cleansed, you should not normally have any trouble here. But babies do get thrush, and this should be treated. Thrush in the mouth looks like milk curds that do not go away between feeds. Apart from being sore for the baby, it does stop him feeding properly and can cause posseting or vomiting. It can happen in the breast-fed baby too, particularly if the mother has had vaginal thrush during pregnancy.

10 Nails

In the first few weeks, your baby's nails will almost certainly need no attention. When they do need cutting, they should be cut straight across and not too short. They must of course be short enough to stop the baby scratching himself. They are very soft at this age and many mothers find that they can trim them better by biting the surplus nail off. In the early weeks the nails often appear to be embedded rather deeply in the surrounding skin and this may even appear inflamed. In nearly every case like this no treatment is required and trying to treat it can, indeed, make matters worse. So if you are worried by the state or appearance of the nails, consult your doctor, but at all costs leave them well alone yourself.

11 The Genitalia and the Foreskin

Many women have doubts and misgivings when they look at this part of their newborn baby, but so often they fail to communicate these doubts to their doctor or midwife. The whole story comes out some months later and a lot of unnecessary worry has been born. Do ask your doctor to check your baby's genitalia if you are worried. I deal here with the most common of the fears.

The opening of the front passage or vagina in a female baby is often covered by a small skin tag which may make it appear that there is no opening. Some female babies have a slight blood loss from the vagina, rather like a small period. This is quite usual and nothing to be alarmed about. It will not recur.

The testicles in a baby boy are usually in the scrotum or sac when they are born, but they need not be there already and may still come down perfectly well of their own accord. If they are not actually in the sack, your doctor may be able to feel them just above the sack and so put your mind at rest. If they still cannot be felt, they should be felt for periodically and, until they are both felt, you should continue to attend your doctor or health clinic regularly. Occasionally they have to be brought down later on.

The foreskin or covering of the penis is there to protect the soft part, or the glans, of the penis. It is supposed to be right over the tip and no attempt should be made to pull it back unless your baby is actually unable to pass water and then no action should be taken except by your doctor. Sometimes the foreskin is so far over the tip that the penis appears very short. This does not matter.

Circumcision goes through phases of being fashionable and unfashionable except, of course, in cases of religious necessity. It is only very rarely a medical necessity. It can, if performed in the presence of any degree of nappy rash, be actually harmful. It is, of course, demanded by some religions and then is usually performed very early and competently. But if your religion does not demand it, there is no need for it unless your baby is unable to pass water without ballooning or swelling of the tip of the penis. Do not be tempted to pull the foreskin back to see if the urethral opening is present. If your baby's nappies are wet you may be sure that all is well and that he is passing water. You should not 'fiddle' with the foreskin for at least the first year, and preferably the second. You will then find that, by gently easing the skin back over the shaft of the penis while the baby is in the bath, the foreskin will slip back easily and smoothly. This will not happen the first time you try it and in fact may take months to accomplish completely, but you will get it back a little further every time you do it. The foreskin is loosely tethered to the shaft of the penis to protect it, and if you pull it back forcefully, you might well cause bleeding to occur and then infection can start up too. If you are in any doubt, of course, do check with your doctor but do not try and force the issue yourself.

Some Common Abnormalities and Worries

1 The Skin

When your baby is first born you will see that he is covered in a waxy greasy substance which has protected him while in the womb. If you do not see him until after he has had his first wash, this might have disappeared. Some babies, particularly those born a little early, may also be covered with a layer of very fine downy hair. This will disappear quite quickly.

You will often notice small white spots on the bridge of the nose and across the cheeks. These are called milia and are due to tiny blocked ducts. They are not infective, are quite normal and need no attention. A dull red mark is often present over the back of the neck. This is called the stork mark (where your baby was delivered by the stork!), it is normal, and in time, it also will go.

There are an enormous variety of birth marks, or naevi, which are commonly seen. Nearly all disappear without treatment, although they may take years rather than months to do so. They need no treatment, but if they do worry you, do discuss this with your doctor. If you have had a forceps delivery, you may see the marks of the forceps on the baby's face. This does not mean the forceps were applied too hard, they will have done the baby no damage and the marks will disappear very rapidly.

118

2 *The Head*

When the baby is being born, the soft bones of the skull are capable of being moulded and pushed so as to come down the birth canal more easily. This moulding often persists after the baby is born and may be very pronounced, giving the baby a high dome-shaped skull. This will all settle down in the first few days and does the baby no harm.

Small swellings under the skin of the scalp are very common. They are called cephalhaematomas and are caused by small collections of blood under the skin. They disappear all by themselves, they do no harm and need cause you no worry.

Do not worry about how much hair your baby has or has not got. Some have none at all when they are born and indeed wait many months before getting any. Some have a little early, lose it and have to start all over again. Some have a great deal and are lucky enough to keep it. This can, I know, be a source of irritation, especially if you have a little girl who is constantly taken for a boy! But do not worry, the speed of growth of the hair seems to have little bearing on the quality of the hair later on.

3 *The Eyes*

In the first few weeks of life a baby often squints—quite suddenly and for no apparent reason his eyes will cross—this is normal and the majority of babies will do it. They will stop doing it within the first two months, usually by six weeks, by which time they are definitely able to focus on you. If a squint persists after this, your doctor should keep a check on it and may then, any time after six months, refer you to the eye specialist at the hospital. The eye specialist himself may well decide just to continue to watch your baby for a while longer, without suggesting any sort of treatment. But having come under his specialist care he will be able to do, or organise, any treatment that is necessary. Whether he advises a patch, glasses, or even an operation will depend so much on the individual squint that it cannot be usefully and fully discussed here. The important thing is to be under expert care early.

Among the commonest mild infections of the very young baby is a sticky eye. This means an inflammation of the eye which causes sticky matter to accumulate and come out of the corner of the eye. If it is associated with a cold then bathing the eye may well be all that is necessary. But if the discharge continues, or there is any sign of redness on the white part, or conjuntiva, of the eye, you should see your doctor for some antibiotic eyedrops.

4 *The Mouth and Tongue Tie*

When your baby is first born and you look into his mouth as he gives his first yawn, you may be startled to see lots of little white spots in the middle of the roof of the mouth. These are not infective and cause no harm. They are called Ebstein's pearls, and they will go.

If the mouth seems to contain milk curds even long after you have fed your baby, it is possible that he has thrush. This is a mild infection caused by a fungus. It should be treated, especially as it often stops a baby feeding properly.

Many mothers are worried about the possibility of tongue tie. True tongue tie—a condition where the tongue cannot be protruded far enough to facilitate normal speech—is very, very uncommon. A short frenulum, however, is quite common. The underside of the tongue is tethered to the floor of the mouth by a thin flap of skin called the frenulum. Usually this is long enough to allow the tongue to be stuck out an inch or so. The tongue needs to be able to reach the lips in order that speech may develop properly. But it does not need to come right out. If the tip of the tongue is tethered down below the level of the lower gum, then this is tongue tie and it does need cutting.

Very occasionally, a baby can be born with a milk tooth, but usually teeth do not start to appear until at least the fifth month.

Swelling of the gums is not a good sign that the tooth is about to erupt. A better sign is when the gum becomes flat on top and a thin grey line appears where the tooth is about to break the surface.

5 Breasts

In the first few days of life the breasts of the baby are often slightly swollen. They may even be a little red. This usually requires no treatment, should be left alone, and will go completely.

6 Clicking Hips

One of the routine tests made by your doctor when your baby is first born is to test the stability of the hip joint. He does this by holding the baby's legs and feeling for the top of the femur, or thigh bone, from behind with his middle finger. He then rotates the leg outwards. He can feel if the rounded end of the femur is securely in the hip joint. He can see if it can be moved freely in and out, or if it is actually outside the joint. There is quite a difference in the degree that an abnormal hip can be rotated outwards. It is surprisingly common, especially in girl babies, to find that the joint is very lax and freely movable, but this should nevertheless continue to be checked to make sure that, in a few weeks, the joint has become firm and stable. If the thigh bone, or femur, is actually outside the hip joint, or if it fails to become stable in a few weeks, the hips must be splinted to avoid damage to the joint. In the very early weeks, the use of a double nappy to keep the legs rotated outwards in a 'frog' position may be all that is necessary in a joint that is just lax. But in a case of actually dislocated hips, it is necessary to splint the legs in plaster. Babies seem to tolerate this remarkably well and in practice it is not nearly so harrowing as it sounds.

It is absolutely vital, however, if your baby has got one or two dislocated hips, that he is treated quickly and adequately. The results of very early treatment can be excellent. But if there is delay long enough to cause damage to the hip joint, it may be a long and tedious problem although much can still be done. I must stress, though, that there is a great difference between hip joints that are dislocatable and those that are actually dislocated.

7 Nails

Nails are very soft and not properly shaped at birth. In fact the toe nails in particular are often very odd indeed, and may appear to be embedded in the skin of the end of the toe. They very rarely require any treatment. Keep them short enough to prevent your baby hurting himself by scratching but otherwise leave them severely alone.

8 Jaundice

Jaundice is the name given to the yellow discoloration of the skin caused by accumulated bile. Normally our livers cope with bile and it is eliminated from the body. But in the newborn baby, the liver machine, as it were, is not working at full capacity. The level of bilirubin, or bile, in the blood stream in all babies rises for the first few days of life. In about a third, or one in three, of all babies, the level of bilirubin rises above 5mg per 100ml and is then visible as a colouring of the skin. Often the first place that it is noticeable is as a yellowing of the nose, especially if you press the nose slightly with your finger and then release it. By the time the level rises to 10mg per 100ml, the whole baby looks slightly yellow.

If the jaudice first appears after the first thirty-six hours and then disappears entirely by the end of the week, there is no cause for alarm. If the jaundice appears earlier than thirty-six hours, then the level of bilirubin must be watched very closely. If the level rises unduly high, it may be necessary to clean the blood of excess bilirubin by exchanging some of the baby's blood for fresh blood. If the jaundice appears within the first twelve hours of life, then it is almost certainly due to blood incompatibility, or the fact that the baby has a different rhesus

122

factor from the mother. This kind of baby will almost certainly need exchange transfusion. The incidence of the particular problem of rhesus incompatibility, however, is very slight compared with ten years ago. This is because a mother who is liable to have babies of a different rhesus factor to her own may be protected from making antibodies, or developing a reaction against that factor, by an injection after delivery of her first baby.

The severe jaundice that is still seen occasionally in the newborn may be due to a widespread infection. A premature baby is more likely to develop a severe jaundice than a full-term one. There are other rare forms of jaundice which will be investigated should the reason for your baby's jaundice not be obvious.

I must stress, however, that by far the majority of cases of jaundice that are noticed by, or pointed out to, worried mothers are those innocent ones which disappear spontaneously and without having become at all severe at any time. So if your baby appears slightly yellow on the third or fourth day, do not worry. It will do him no harm apart from, possibly, temporarily slowing him down in feeding.

9 Sternomastoid Tumour

I mention this here and separately not because of its importance or severity from a medical point of view, but because of the anguish it can cause through misunderstanding. It is not a tumour. It is not a growth of any sort. It is in fact a bruise, or small collection of blood, in the muscle of the neck. It causes a swelling which stops the baby moving his head freely to that side. The baby therefore has a rather stiff one-sided look. It is in no way damaging and in time it will disappear.

10 Nerve Damage at Birth

If it has been necessary for you to have a forceps delivery, and if this has proved a bit difficult, it is possible that some temporary damage can be done to the baby as it is being born. This can result in a temporary loss of function. Nerves make the muscles work and if the nerves are squeezed during delivery, the muscles will not work properly. This can happen with the nerves that supply the muscles of the face, and then the face can appear to droop on one side. Sometimes the muscles of the arm can be affected and the arm will appear to hang rather limply.

These conditions very rarely last more than a few days after birth, and there will not be any permanent damage.

11 Ears

Ears can be an extraordinary variety of shapes when the baby is first born and, because they are so soft, they can be bent into even odder shapes. It is not unusual to find extra pieces of skin or flaps around the ears. These need no attention at first and, unless they are unsightly, they need not be touched. They have no bearing on the efficiency of the ear.

Many ears appear to stick out unduly and it is all too easy to let the ear fold the wrong way when the baby is lying down. Do make sure that the ear is folded flat against the head when your baby goes off to sleep. Sticking the ears back with Elastoplast will not affect the degree that the ears stick out and can, indeed, cause soreness. I think that you will achieve as much by carefully laying the ear flat in the early days as you will by using sticking plaster, and you will certainly avoid the possibility of causing infection behind the ear—a notoriously difficult place to keep clean anyway in the early days! Any degree of sticking out that is worse than this will do better with proper medical treatment. Sticking out of the ears or 'bat ears' bears no relationship whatsoever to the intelligence of the child.

12 Undescended Testicles and Circumcision

I have dealt with this subject fairly fully in a previous section, but I will make the important points once again.

Circumcision is very rarely medically necessary. It is an operation that can have side effects and should not be carried out unnecessarily. The foreskin is present in a very young baby in order to protect the delicate skin of the penis and is, in fact, tethered to the shaft of the penis by strands of tissue. If you force the foreskin back too early you break these adhesions and may cause bleeding and infection. During the second year of life, the foreskin may be gently eased back while the baby is in the bath. This is the same movement as slipping the finger part of a glove on to the finger.

Testicles are usually in the scrotum, or sack, at birth. If they are not fully descended at birth they may be anywhere between the abdomen, where they originally formed, and down the canal through which they travel to reach the scrotum. Sometimes it is necessary to do an operation in order to bring the testicle down, but your doctor may well be able to reassure you that he can feel the testicles just above the scrotum from where they will usually come down on their own. Finally, remember that one testicle is just as adequate as two when it comes to having children in later life. However, although this is true, you should continue to attend your doctor if only one testicle appears.

13 *Talipes*

Babies are sometimes born with their feet turning inwards or, less commonly, outwards. If the abnormality is mild, then all that is necessary is physiotherapy and exercises. If the condition is more severe, then further treatment such as splinting may be necessary. As with so many things in young babies, the tissues and bones are easily manipulated because they are so soft. And therefore, if these conditions are recognised and treated early, the results are often extremely good.

14 *Umbilical Hernia*

In some babies the muscles that form the wall of the front of the stomach are not tightly closed together. This can cause a small protrusion, or hernia, which makes the umbilicus, or tummy button, look larger than it should, and also to enlarge on coughing. This condition, provided that the protrusion is small, requires no interference and will most often right itself during the first few years of life. No hernia will be improved by strapping a penny over it! This is an old wives' tale!

15 Vomiting and Posseting

Babies often regurgitate or bring up fluid and mucus in the first twenty-four hours. If this continues and is associated with the failure of the motion to become a normal colour, then it can mean that there is an obstruction in the intestine. This is rare, and many babies do continue to bring up small amounts of fluid with wind which can be annoying but, provided that the motion is normal, and the baby thrives, it need give no cause for anxiety. It is, of course, even more important to put your baby to sleep on his side or stomach if he does have this tendency to posset.

There are actual structural abnormalities which will cause a baby to vomit, but these are usually obvious in that the vomiting is consistent, severe, and the baby is unhappy and does not thrive. Provided that your baby is happy, sleeps fairly well and grows, there is unlikely to be much wrong. There are faults in feeding and winding routine that can cause this posseting, but they are fully dealt with in the section on feeding. Having said that, there are undoubtedly babies who will continue to regurgitate a little at every feed for no apparent reason.

If your baby suddenly starts to vomit when he has not done so before, this can be a more serious sign and you should check with your doctor. Or if he has always tended to bring up a little and suddenly starts to bring up a lot, it is again wise to check with your doctor.

There is a condition called pyloric stenosis in which a baby suddenly starts to vomit copiously at every feed. The vomiting is known as 'projectile', because it shoots out and may land on the floor several feet away from where you are feeding. This is due to an enlarged muscle valve at the end of the stomach sac, which contracts violently and forces the feed back up out of the stomach. This condition requires an operation to cure it, but the results of this operation are excellent. The condition is commonest in first-born boys.

Finally, at any age, including the first week of life, a baby can have a stomach upset or infection which will be accompanied by vomiting. Vomiting and diarrhoea caused by a stomach upset are severe symptoms in a young baby and should be treated promptly. Vomiting, in fact, is a very common symptom accompanying an infection in any part of the body.

The important thing, therefore, is to take note of any change in your baby's habits. Habitual posseting is not in itself of much importance, provided that the baby is thriving, but the sudden onset of vomiting in a previously normal baby is always of importance and you should seek advice soon.

16 *Neonatal Convulsions or Twitching*

Some babies, in the first week of life, may be seen to twitch periodically or, in its grosser form, to actually have a small convulsion. This must be reported, even if you are still in hospital with your baby, as you may have been the only person to have seen it. The two commonest causes for this are (a) low blood sugar, particularly in a low birth-weight baby, and (b) a low blood calcium level. Both conditions are readily tested and comparatively easily treated. They are self-limiting as the baby grows and will not last. Convulsions which occur with a high temperature in later infancy are dealt with in a later section.

17 *Respiratory or Breathing Difficulties*

These are the commonest difficulties which occur during the first few days of a baby's life. They are more common in babies who have had difficult deliveries, in premature babies, babies of low birth-weight, and those of diabetic mothers. The exact cause of the particular illness called respiratory distress is not clear, but the baby breathes more rapidly than usual, is seen to draw in his chest wall in the effort to breathe and cannot maintain a good healthy pink colour. He cannot feed properly and may have to be fed by a tube. He will probably need to be nursed in an incubator. The condition may only last a day or so, particularly if it has been caused by a difficult delivery, but in a premature baby it may last longer and become a cause for anxiety.

This section seems like a long list of possible difficulties and abnormalities. It is important to realise that the vast majority of babies have few, if any, of them. It is very important to recognise those that are not severe and to be able to reassure yourself that they will go. There are many other small things that you may notice which can cause extreme anxiety if you keep them to yourself. I would stress that you must tell your doctor or midwife of any worries that you have. When you have just had a baby, you will often spend hours just observing him. You may notice something that nobody else has pointed out to you. Very often it is of no consequence at all, and it may, indeed, be absolutely normal, but it can be magnified in your mind if you do not discuss it with someone else. Very often they will be able to reassure you completely.

The Normal Newborn Child

The commonest question asked by nearly every mother when her baby is first born is 'Is he all right?' The preceding sections deal with most of the actual physical things that you will notice. This section explains how he should react and what he can or cannot be expected to do.

The normal newborn baby sleeps most of the time. When he is not actually sleeping, he is usually crying. He will often be crying for a feed, will be fed and then, satisfied, will fall asleep again. He may, of course, cry because he is uncomfortable and, later on, he may cry because he is dirty or wet. Sudden noise will startle and often distress him. Amazingly early he will learn to cry, or at least whimper, when he is put down to sleep after being cuddled. Do not be misled into picking him up again too soon. If he is well fed and dry then at least give him the chance to settle again to sleep.

Reflexes Present in the Normal Newborn Baby

These are instinctive movements that all babies will make in response to certain touches. If you stroke your baby's cheek gently he will turn his head towards the stroking finger. This is called the rooting reflex and represents the baby turning to find the nipple and his next feed.

If you make a sudden loud noise, or startle your baby, he will jerk both his hands together up above his head and then bring them back together as though he was cuddling something to him. This is called the startle, or Moro, reflex.

If you touch your baby's foot lightly against a table top while supporting his body, he will make walking movements with his legs. If you touch the top of his foot under the edge of a table he will lift the leg on to the table as though he were stepping up, although of course he cannot, and should not, put any weight on his legs. These are appropriately the walking, or stepping, reflexes.

If you rub your finger gently over the palm of your baby's hand he will grasp it firmly. He can often actually be lifted up this way although of course you cannot safely assume that his grasp will be strong enough for this.

Finally, there is what is called the 'tonic neck reflex'. This means that when you turn your baby's head to the right, the right arm and the right leg will stretch out and the left arm and left leg will flex, or bend, up. Conversely, if you turn your baby's head to the left, then the left arm and left leg extend and the right arm and leg will flex up.

These are the earliest primitive reflexes by which your doctor will tell that your baby is 'working' normally. They are only present for the first three months of life.

During the first few weeks your baby will sleep with his legs drawn up under him and usually with his hands gently closed, too. He will sleep most of the time and will usually be crying when he is awake. If you place him face downwards in his cot he will usually turn his head automatically to one side, but if you hold him in a sitting position he cannot support his own head which will flop forwards. At all times you must support his head at this stage. He has no control over it and if you hold him face downwards, his head will drop unsupported between his shoulders. While sitting, his whole back, neck and head are one round curve.

In spite of this lack of muscle tone, however, he has quite a range of facial movements and expressions, even at this very early stage. He can yawn in a most adult way. He can sneeze and cough. He can, of course, bring up his wind and can even hiccup. He will not be able to smile during the first month, but will show gradually increasing awareness of his surroundings. He will be absorbed by, and may even turn towards, the bright light of a window, and will blink his eyes tight shut if a bright light is shone too near them suddenly.

The Six-week Check

Your doctor or clinic will arrange to give your baby a complete physical examination at this stage.

He will by now be definitely aware of his surroundings. He will be soothed by the sound of his mother's voice close by. He will not, however, stop screaming if he is really hungry—reassurance only goes so far! He will have started to focus on your face and will observe you with an unblinking stare if you rest him on your lap and talk to him. He can certainly appreciate light and brightness at some distance, but can focus on objects at only about six inches. This distance will gradually increase. He will often, at this stage, be able to follow an object or light through an arc in front of his eyes but not right round to the sides. He will have begun to make little noises by this time. And most rewarding of all he will have started to smile at you. There will be many heated arguments as to whether it is a smile or wind when it first appears! Most babies are smiling by six weeks but there is no doubt that some do smile as early as four weeks. Under a month I am usually inclined to think that it is wind. The expression in your baby's eyes will change when he really smiles at you. And whenever it does come it is certainly rewarding. You are sometimes feeling, by this time, that having a baby is a constant round of feeding, changing and sleeping with little reward! Almost daily now he will learn new tricks and new responses and it will be harder and harder to limit the cuddle and play time so that he has adequate rest.

The Three-month Check

By now your baby is really responding to you. He loves to watch your face intently while you talk to him. He will smile delightedly while you play with him, or gently tickle him. He will watch you from his cot while you move around.

He will by now be trying to hold a rattle for a few seconds, although he will not be able to hold on to it for long, his arm will suddenly jerk across his face, he will lose the rattle and will often hit himself in the process.

He will still be startled by sudden loud noise, but will quite definitely turn his head towards interesting noises. He will now be getting quite excited when he can see a feed being prepared and will learn to show his frustration at being kept waiting. He will be quite crafty enough to cry when put back to bed, hoping that he will be picked up again. Beware that your baby does not start to rule you! He very easily can, even at this early stage. You will save yourself so much anxiety and difficulty if you are gentle but firm at this stage.

Your baby is becoming much more active now. If his legs are free he will kick out strongly and will open and close his arms. His movements are wild and jerky. Sometimes they will even appear purposeful. He will begin to play with his own hands and to watch them in front of his face. Towards the end of the three months he will show an extraordinary sign which is quite fascinating to watch. This is called 'hand regard' and he will stare at his own arm or outstretched hand unmoving and un-blinking. Not all babies do this for any length of time, but if they do it can be quite unnerving, so still are they.

He is much less floppy now and when held in a sitting position will be able to hold his head erect for a few seconds before it drops forwards. If you hold him face downwards he will be able to keep his head at the same level as his shoulders and, although you must continue to support his head at all times, he will feel much firmer to handle. If you actually lay him down on the floor, face downwards, he will be able to lift his head and the top part of his chest for a few seconds. Babies who habitually sleep on their stomachs, rather than on their backs, seem to develop this ability more quickly.

People often ask for guidelines as to intelligence in their child. There are few, if any, foolproof methods of assessing intelligence at this early stage. Possibly those babies who smile really earlier than normal and those who speak earlier than normal are likely to be intelligent. But, apart from these two signs to which there are plenty of exceptions, as proved later in life, there is no other reliable test at this age.

Play in the Early Months

These first few months are, in many ways, very difficult, especially as the baby gets to about three months. He is not physically capable of amusing himself, but needs to be amused or he becomes bored very quickly. To be taken out in a pram or car is, of course, ideal entertainment from your baby's point of view. There is a never-ending change of scene, with different

132

colours and shapes, and yet he has to do little else but turn his head to watch.

It is difficult to achieve this moving, interesting environment indoors. You will probably receive many rattles from kind relatives, especially if it is your first baby. Many of these will not be suitable for his very early grasp. Try to find a rattle that has a small enough ring or handle for him to grasp, is a bright enough colour to be interesting, and with a musical enough noise not to be irritating or deafening for either of you. I have found that a piece of string, hung between two chairs over a coloured rug on which your baby can play, is an excellent means of ringing the changes. You can hang all sorts of interesting objects and shapes over the string. This is easy to erect, easy to dismantle and can be varied every day. My children have always enjoyed a variety of kitchen equipment dangling and rattling about, just as much as an expensive toy. Do make sure that the noises you produce are not too loud and are at least a little musical. And, of course, the objects that you use must be safe and not liable to injure your baby in any way.

Mobiles are delightful things to hang above your baby's cot. They may well provide an interesting enough environment to keep him amused for some while when he first awakes. There are countless very attractive mobiles that you can buy, but you do not have to spend any money at all. Pictures cut out from magazines and pasted on to card do very well. I have made mobiles from such diverse objects as fir cones, egg boxes, tin foil (making superb fish) and even just coloured pieces of paper cut into interesting shapes. The gummed paper squares that you can buy from most toy shops are in beautifully bright colours and save you having to do any other sticking. They do not have to be complicated or clever. All they need to be is bright and moving. Obviously the lighter the mobile the better it will move.

I think that it is unwise to leave any toys in the cot at this age. I must admit that I do not even like any toys strung across

133

the cot at this time, especially while the baby is sleeping. Furry toys are definitely not a good idea as nearly all young babies suck anything that they can reach. I would leave the cot uncluttered at this earliest stage and just make the outside environment attractive. Play is for very short periods at this time and should be supervised if at all possible.

Finally, there is play in the bath. A flotilla of plastic ducks, especially if one of them has a bell in it, is all that is required at this stage. But the bath does tend to be rather 'taken over' by children's toys later on, if you are not careful. An excellent idea that I inherited is to have a plastic shopping-bag hung above the bath into which all the dripping toys can be placed. This keeps them out of adults' way and enables them to drip safely into the bath while they are still wet.

Early Psychology of the Newborn Baby in the Family

There is no doubt that a newborn baby is a tremendous upheaval in a family, both physically and emotionally. In many ways we are not very well equipped to cope with it during the early months, simply because we are overtired from short nights. In this rather bad state of frayed nerves, it is all too easy to let irritation and bad temper get the upper hand to spoil the new experience.

The first thoughts of both husband and wife will be for the new baby. He is new and he is helpless. But you must not forget that you both have to continue to care for each other just as much as you did before the baby arrived. There are at least three new relationships that must be established. Husband and wife have to re-establish a new relationship. Mother and father have to establish a relationship with the baby. And perhaps most important and most difficult, your other children, if you have any, must accept and welcome the new baby. It is all too easy to forget all this in the excitement and tiredness of coping with a demanding new member of the family. There do not seem to be any hard and fast rules as to which children will show jealousy of the new arrival. Most children seem to accept him at first. He is a novelty, quite fun to watch and there are new things to learn. But, after a few weeks or so, they suddenly seem to realise that the novelty is here to stay.

The most important general rule to remember is to really try and involve your older child and, however much it may slow you up, try to find some things in which he can be important in looking after the new arrival. Do try and involve your older child at feeding time, which is when many jealousies first seem to arise. And do try and keep some part of every day free for your older child to have your undivided attention. Your baby will, hopefully, be sleeping for long periods. Try and keep one of these times free for special play with another child. It is unwise, as a general rule, to start an older child off at play school or school proper just at the moment when the new baby arrives home. Sometimes it is unavoidable, but if there can be a settling-in period for fathers, mothers, babies and older children, it usually pays off. Once jealousy creeps in, in any member of the family, it is much more difficult to reassure them. In spite of your own tiredness, and often temporary anxiety, it is really worth the extra effort to try and make sure that nobody suddenly feels left out. One of the most difficult things to cope with is the natural desire of older children to pick up and cuddle young babies. You must let them hold the baby. You just have to make sure that he is held safely.

If you have thought about the problem during your pregnancy, you will have done much to prepare the older children for the arrival. Do not forget that, for them, the waiting period will have seemed interminable. And the actual arrival often seems an anti-climax, with mother short tempered and over-tired. I have found that to reserve a special time for older children, once the baby has been settled after his 5 or 6 pm feed, is invaluable. Bedtime for the older child can then proceed along the old established routine.

It often helps to prepare you and your husband's supper earlier in the day. It is in the early evening that your energy will often seem to run out completely, and there is nothing that you feel like less than preparing another meal. Whatever your husband's hours of work, and even if you have up to now had a high tea together at about six, I cannot agree that to try and feed a baby, a toddler and yourselves at the same time is a good idea. Someone will not have a peaceful and adequate meal and it will nearly always be you and sometimes your husband as well, and, I am afraid to say, often all of you. Besides which, it is most agreeable, at some time in the day, to have a peaceful adult meal without having to supervise anyone and where perhaps your conversation can be other than of the baby.

Do not be afraid to alter your bedtime temporarily to suit your baby's feed time. There is many an evening, during the first few weeks, that I have gone to bed as early as seven or eight just to catch up on a few hour's sleep. And if it is your first baby, do not be ashamed to take a morning or afternoon sleep with him. This period of frequent feeds and sleepless nights soon passes, although at the time it appears to go on for ever.

It is really worthwhile trying to establish the relationships and routine early on. Of course if you have older children, who perhaps need to be taken to school, you will not necessarily be able to establish the most restful routine for a newborn baby. But you can still find some routine and, remember, you can usually alter one part of the day's schedule but rarely two without upsetting your baby's sleep pattern.

Admittedly the discussion above is a very generalised one. It must be, because every child reacts individually and indeed every family unit will react individually. I would never quarrel with any routine or any approach to a particular problem if it works. But a conscious effort there certainly needs to be, and a routine there must be, if your life is to be comparatively peaceful. Your rewards will be great if you can achieve a peaceful and harmonious enlarged family unit.

136

PART FOUR

YOUR GROWING CHILD

Further Things You Will Need

1 *The Cot*

If you have not already invested in your cot, you must do so at this stage. No baby will sleep well if he is cramped. The carry-cot may still be quite adequate for his daytime sleep, but at night he must be free to move about and change his position. I have already discussed points to be watched for in buying a cot in a previous section.

2 *Chairs and Highchairs*

There are basically three types of chairs available on the market. There is the sling, or hammock, type of baby rocking chair. These have a limited use in that, as soon as your baby can pull himself up to a sitting position, he will not be safe in the chair. But they do fulfil, in my opinion, the needs of the very young baby, that is from six weeks to six months. A baby should not be put into a chair with an upright back until he is able to support his own back.

Secondly, there are chairs which double as highchairs with an upright back which can be put into a reclining position. This is excellent, but it still cannot be used as early as the hammock support type above. But it can, of course, go on being used long after the hammock cannot and can often also be used as a conventional highchair as long as the baby's bottom is small enough to fit into it; or of course until he becomes too strong for it. Some have attachments for hooking over an ordinary upright dining chair.

Then, thirdly and finally, there is the ordinary, conventional, rigid highchair made of plastic or wood which can often be used first, as a highchair, and then lowered to be used with a small table, or its own attached table, as a nursery feeding chair.

It is not many of us these days who can happily afford all three types of chair which would take us safely from six weeks to toddler stage. The combination that we choose obviously depends upon individual preference. I have always enjoyed having the hammock chair for my babies, simply because it answers that very early requirement when your baby is old enough to enjoy watching you while you do something, but before he can sit, or indeed lie, long enough to do so. There is no doubt that even a very young baby can become bored and, if he is bright and alert, then his mental development and need for entertainment seems to outstrip his physical development. So, this hammock type of seat, which enables him to be entertained without strain from a very early age, seems to be invaluable.

Once he is ready to sit upright in a more conventional chair, then convenience and cost are greater factors to take into account. Some of the adaptable chairs which turn into a reclining seat, a swing, or a high chair do certainly amuse a baby, but they are more finicky and on the whole less substantial than the conventional highchair. My advice would be to shop around. See what your friends use and listen to their praises and grumbles.

3 *Pushchairs*

Here the variety is enormous and for every type there seems to be so much to be said that it can be very difficult to make up your mind. There are, again, three main choices. You can buy a substantial pushchair with a hood which is large enough for your baby to sleep in. You can buy a lightweight pushchair which will not be adaptable for sleeping in, but which will be infinitely easier to carry around. And, finally, you can buy a baby-buggy type of chair whose greater advantage is its lightness and ease of folding and packing. For each parent one of these considerations is more important than the others. There are no real hazards to any of them, except that I do think the baby-buggy should be used with caution for the very young. I feel that a baby-buggy type of chair should not be used unless your baby can sit up unsupported, and this usually means nearer nine months than six. Of course you cannot use the conventional pushchair until your baby can sit up anyway, but there is a tendency simply because the baby can be propped in a buggy, to take him out in a pushchair before he is ready.

4 *Clothing*

Underwear remains basically the same design throughout baby-hood and into childhood. The same criteria exist. You should have cotton vests for the summer, although you do not have to put your baby in a vest then, especially if our summers continue to be so extraordinarily hot. You should have wool vests for the winter. I can see no sense in buying very small sizes at all as the width of the items changes very little. It is merely the length that alters. So why not get a good long vest while you are about it, it will last longer.

Many mothers keep their babies in Babygros throughout the first year and even well into the second. Of course they make ideal garments at night, but I like to ring the changes during the day. If you have a little girl it is such fun to start finding little dresses and tights to match and there is a beautiful selection of romper suits, dungarees and playclothes for boys and girls. If this is your first baby you may well find, as I did, that dungarees can be easily adapted for boys and girls so that they can be used for your second child even if it is a different sex. The main reason why children's clothing can prove such an expense is that the children grow so fast that they never get complete wear out of any garment. So if you can possibly find clothes that will suit a boy or girl, I think it is well worth it. Of course, you must have one or two beautiful female outfits if you have a little girl, but do remember that dresses for a one year old make beautiful smock tops for a three to four year old.

If you can, stick to pure cotton or pure wool next to the skin. A baby's skin is very sensitive and, as I have explained in a previous chapter, they are very likely to get spots if they become sweaty. Nylon certainly seems to make a baby more sweaty and should be avoided, at first, next to the skin. Later on, many children seem to tolerate it very well, although my personal preference remains for cotton where possible. Certainly, in the summer, pure cotton dresses are infinitely more cooling than nylon, although admittedly you do have to iron them.

It is astonishingly difficult to find jerseys that really fit. If they are long enough in the body they are invariably too long in the sleeve and if the sleeve is correct then you are lucky if the Jersey reaches the waist! If you are faced with this choice, then get the too long sleeves! At least your baby will be warm! In the same way, tights that have adequate leg length seem to have enough panty to stretch to the shoulder and a fitting panty part in fact drops to the knees because the legs are far too short. Amongst all these frustrations I would stress that you should get upper and lower garments that overlap really well. And for the toddler a play suit or dungarees are infinitely preferable to trousers which, you will find, rarely stay on. Do buy your playsuit too long in the leg. You can always turn the legs up initially but you cannot lengthen them when they no longer reach your baby's ankles. In contrast to vests, dresses and T-shirts, these playsuits or dungarees are better bought in synthetic fibres. Firstly, they will not have to be ironed, secondly, they stretch better to allow freer movement and, thirdly, they require no special washing routine.

Your baby is now, hopefully, clothed in underwear and indoor clothing. There remains outdoor clothing to be bought. I have always bought anoraks in preference to coats at this young age, partly because by combining warmth with waterproofing it is cheaper and, secondly, because they are more easily handed down to your next child. There is nothing more snug than those beautiful all-in-one suits during the first two years and, if you can possibly afford one, then do make sure that it is washable—toddlers are amazingly dirty! Of course it is marvellous to have rainproof clothing as well, but all the clothes you buy at this stage will be usable for such a short time that I really do not think it is a justifiable expense. There are marvel-

142

lous all-in-one mackintosh covers for pushchairs which, I think, are much more convenient to use than re-dressing a toddler in yet another suit of clothing.

5 Shoes

Finally, there comes the vexed question of shoes. You should not buy firm walking shoes until your baby has been walking properly for at least a month. A baby can learn to walk perfectly well without shoes and, indeed, should do so. It is not until he has been walking a little while that his feet will assume a true walking shape. If you buy hard shoes prematurely, you might cramp his feet while they are changing shape. So wait until he is walking well before you buy and when you do, go to a shop, specialising in children's shoes, which has a machine to measure the length and the breadth of his feet accurately. There is no reason, of course, why you should not protect your baby's feet with soft shoes while he is crawling and these should err on the side of being too large rather than fitting, and should be made entirely of soft material.

The cost of children's shoes is phenomenal and your subequent buying will often be dictated by cost. However, I am sure it is worth getting that first pair of shoes of good material and fitting properly. Once your child's feet have formed, subsequent pairs of shoes need not be so expensive, provided that certain rules are followed. They must be flat. They must be wide enough, and do not forget that toes fan out when you tread down. They must not cramp or pinch at any point. And, finally, they must be long enough. It is far better to have shoes too large than too small. If you can manage it, buy leather uppers, they are far superior to plastic. I have always found buckles easier to manage in the early years than laces. The latter are constantly coming undone and tripping the child up. The former are less easy to undo and therefore the shoes are removed less often. Wellington boots are marvellous for outdoor winter use, but do remember that your toddler will very often lose them in the mud or take them off to examine them. Your washing will then have increased again.

6 *Reins*

Although I am, in principle, against tethering, tying or otherwise restraining children, there are definitely occasions when reins are essential. An active toddler will need reins in his high chair—for your peace of mind as much as for his safety. Again, an active toddler will need reins in his pushchair. And, initially, when he starts to walk, instead of being in a pushchair, if you are in a built-up area, you really must use reins. It takes but a split second for your child to leave your side and step into the road. But, as freedom is so much better if it can be managed, do try and find some time for walking in a park or field, where he can be free just to toddle at will. And, however much he may resent it, do keep his reins on all the time that he might be in danger.

Finally I must mention the other toys and apparatus which are used increasingly. The main two are the baby-bouncer and the baby-walker.

There is no doubt that baby-bouncers do give a great deal of pleasure to a lot of infants if used correctly. But they should not be used for long periods, children should not be left in them and they must not be used too young. My personal view is that for the length of time they can be safely and wisely used, they are unnecessary. I believe that a baby can and will develop from the floor. He will do his own bouncing when he has learnt to stand holding on to chairs. I do not believe that you should ever force the pace in a child's physical development unless you are expressly advised to do so. I do not believe in 'lazy children' except in very exceptional circumstances. So let your baby develop naturally. By all means applaud and encourage him when he learns a new skill, but do not try to make him stand or walk before he is ready to do so.

Similarly, I can see little advantage in baby-walkers in children who are developing normally. They are of enormous value in certain circumstances, where development is slow, or in the case of certain handicaps. A baby-walker here might be actively advised. But a child who goes through all the normal stages of sitting, crawling or squirming, standing and then walking does not need these sorts of artificial aids. A wheeled walking toy, of course, is of enormous value when your toddler is learning to walk, but even here my children have pushed their own pushchairs along with quite as much, if not more, enjoyment than the toys provided for that purpose.

I will discuss the development of children at greater length in a later section, but it is worthwhile saying here that, in spite of the normal ages of development that we are all so fond of quoting, children do develop at remarkably different rates. And no amount of worrying or buying of special equipment will influence this development at all. If you are worried that your baby is slow to stand or walk, do check with your doctor for a physical defect, but if there is none, then be content to sit back, encourage and enjoy.

Feeding and Weaning

I have already stated in the first part of this book that no child needs solid food until he is not satisfied with an 8oz bottle. There are a few exceptions to this rule, as there must be to all rules, but they are few. With the majority of children this means starting solid food between the third and the sixth month. Whenever you start to wean your child, the art is to do it slowly and gradually. Solid food must be introduced really slowly; at one meal only at first and one type of food at a time. I have always made it a rule never to introduce more than one new food a day. And in the first month of weaning I have never introduced more than one new food in a week. There will be foods that are much less well tolerated than others and, by introducing new foods really gradually, you can isolate any that cause trouble. Many people, for instance, find that their small children cannot tolerate carrots and that any carrot-containing mixture will give the baby loose motions. So try and be systematic about your weaning; getting your baby used to and enjoying one new taste at a time.

The following discussion on weaning, therefore, consists of general rules rather than special diets.

1 Introduce the first solid food at one meal only, preferably during the day, so that if it causes colic you will not be up all night.

2 Introduce a plain cereal first, eg Farex.

3 Give a very small quantity initially, ie one level teaspoonful of powdered cereal made up with a little sugar and milk.

4 Do make the mixture sufficiently fluid. Babies do not like a solid spongy mass.

5 Do make sure it is warm; and here a warming plate with hot water underneath does help.

6 Do not think that because your baby spits he does not like it. All babies spit before they have learned to eat off a spoon.

7 Depress the spoon lightly on the baby's tongue and let him suck off the spoon.

8 Do check the temperature of the food. He will be greatly put off solid food if at the first attempt he gets a burnt tongue.

Individual babies vary a great deal as to the best time to give the solid food. For some their thirst is so great that you must allow them to have some part of their milk feed before their solids. For others, if you allow them to have part of their milk feed first, they will not be content until they have finished it. Most babies will be too full at the end of a milk feed to bother about trying a new and less rewarding type of feeding. For myself, I have always favoured a little of the milk feed first to quench the thirst, solids next, and then finishing up with the rest of the milk feed.

Your baby is now, hopefully, taking a little cereal at one feed. Now you can introduce it at another feed, preferably the evening one. Do not be afraid that cereal will make him fat, it is the quantity of the feed given that will make the baby too fat. But, knowing that your baby tolerates a milky cereal, you can now introduce another food, such as lightly boiled egg yolk. Do not give the white of the egg. Babies seem to like the soft yolk and a teaspoonful of egg yolk represents a considerable increase in your baby's diet. Once you have seen this tolerated and, indeed, enjoyed, you can introduce another food. Always keep the quantity right down; a teaspoonful is quite sufficient at this early stage. And I would suggest making the midday meal the experimental one and the evening meal the milky cereal which is readily digested and unlikely to give trouble at night.

Your aim during this weaning period, that is roughly from three to nine months, is to get your child, eventually, onto the three solid meals a day, at times that suit your schedule. You should continue to give milk in the morning and last thing at night, although fruit drinks can replace the other daytime feeds.

I would suggest that you give solid food in roughly the order below, not introducing more than one major new taste in the week:

a) cereals made up with milk
b) egg yolk
c) fruit purées
d) vegetable purées
e) vegetable purées with gravy
f) meat purées

There are a large number of cereal powders, often fortified with vitamins, that are very easily digested, easily made up with boiled milk and which can be used as a vehicle for introducing new foods. For instance, apple purée can be added to Farex and, indeed, the Farex itself can be made up with other liquids.

If you are lucky enough to have a liquidiser, then you can make up your own puréed foods, although the quantities that you must use do sometimes make this wasteful. I have puréed vegetables, given a little to the baby and used the remainder very satisfactorily as a basis for soup.

But, in the absence of a liquidiser, the numerous baby purées in jars or cans are an excellent substitute, and of course they are very convenient. You can also use half one day and safely save the remainder in a refrigerator for the next day.

However you do decide to manage this stage of weaning, do watch out for particular foods which are not well tolerated. Many babies cannot tolerate carrots, and other green vegetables in excess can be a problem. I have repeatedly found that meats given in purée form are the least well tolerated of the proteins and should be introduced last in the weaning table.

Fruit should be fresh, or used from baby tins, or jars and you should not use the syrup fruit tins as they are too sugary.

Throughout this period your baby should continue with at least a pint of milk in one form or another. A vitamin C concentrated fruit drink such as Ribena or Delrosa should be a definite part of the day's menu. Too much of these fruit drinks however, do sometimes increase the baby's sugar intake too much. If this does happen, you will find that your baby tends to have loose motions.

If you are using your own liquidiser to make up your baby's first foods then, as the months go by, you can liquidise them less thoroughly and therefore get him used to a slightly more 'bitty' texture. If using the tins or jars from Heinz, Gerber or Robinson, you will find that these are graded from a fine texture to a more 'bitty' one.

At any rate, by the time your baby is ready to sit in his highchair, to wait for his food, he will begin to enjoy holding onto something that he can chew. Rusks form an excellent beginning and I find the harder ones such as Ovaltine teething rusks safer, because the baby is less likely to be able to break a bit off and choke on it. He will have to suck at it. You should be with your baby all the time that he has food in his hand. It is all too easy for him to choke if a larger piece does get broken off, and if he should choke, do not wait. Turn him upside down and pull out the food with your finger.

By the time that he is eight or nine months you can substitute the soft adult cereals, such as Weetabix, for the baby cereals. A banana mashed finely with sugar and a little milk will often be greatly enjoyed. And you can start experimenting with all sorts of different tastes. If you discover something that he definitely seems to dislike, do not persevere. Forget all about it and then try again in a month or so. Surprisingly, very young babies seem to love the taste of cheese, although I have found that they cannot often tolerate it cooked. Whatever you try, do make sure that it is never given too hot. If a baby burns his tongue on a new food he will not recognise that it is the heat that has upset him, only that the food, whatever it was, caused him pain. I have seen several babies put off scrambled eggs for months because, although it cools very rapidly on the outside, it tends to retain its heat in the middle.

By the time your baby is reaching the end of his first year, he will be able to eat most of what you are cooking for the rest of the family, provided that it is not too highly flavoured. Meat remains a problem the longest, because it cannot be mashed up finely enough. A joint can be scraped to form a meat purée and liver can be mashed very finely. But you will have to continue to liquidise most other forms of meat.

One of the other foods so often left out, and one which is most nutritious, is fish. It is best to cook or steam it in milk and you can be fairly sure that the tail end of filleted fish will have no bones in it. This fish, mashed with potato and milk makes a very nourishing and enjoyable alternative to his diet.

Tea is often a problem meal and many of us tend to produce eggs in one form or another every day. This is fine for the baby nutritionally, but there is no doubt that children, and even young babies, can become bored with the same diet day after day. So, it is best to ring the changes if you can. I have found that tea consisting mainly of biscuits and cakes produces a prodigious

thirst in my children which makes them drink excessively afterwards and, of course, then they tend to soak the bed. If you can
leave over some custard or rice pudding or any of the numerous
and excellent packet puddings to be made up with milk, then it
does help to fill them up at tea time without drying them up.
Also children are very tired by teatime, and eating heavy or
stodgy food is an effort. Although the children will be hungry,
they often need to be coaxed somewhat to eat sufficient to
enable them to sleep really soundly. A baby who has insufficient
to eat at teatime will not sleep so well. Of course, throughout
most of the first year, the last meal of the day will remain warm
milk, but later on a soft milk pudding will go down infinitely
easier than a large sticky bun which he will often push impatiently
away.

From the sixth month onwards, it is wise to start encouraging
him to take drinks from a cup rather than a bottle. Start off with
the fruit drink in mid morning. Let him have his hands round the
cup himself. Do not force him to accept a cup too quickly, he
will soon manage very well on his own. Amongst some mothers,
it seems to be a point of honour to get their babies to use an
adult cup before their friends' babies. I see no virtue in such a
race and believe that the weaning from bottle to cup should be
very gradual. I have absolutely no objections to the use of baby-
cups. These are lidded cups with a spout. They are much easier
for the baby to manage at first and have the added advantage
that when dropped accidentally there is little or no mess on your
carpet. Or even more important, perhaps, on your friends'
carpets. I do not believe that using these baby-cups will stop
your child developing quickly. The cups, however, should be
used for drinking at a set time and the child should not be allowed to wander round using the cup as a kind of dummy.
And, while I heartily endorse the use of these cups, particularly
when you are out, I would also encourage the use of an ordinary
cup in the safety of your own kitchen. I usually start the two
simultaneously. I would encourage the use of an ordinary cup

whenever time and place allow it, but continue to use a baby-cup whenever I am out and, indeed, find them invaluable in cars while travelling, even well into the baby's second and third year.

But, drinking apart, do encourage your child to feed himself whenever you can. Very early on he will recognise his spoon as the instrument of feeding. I know only too well how irritating it is to find half his dinner on the floor and how much easier it is to restrain his flailing arms and spoon his dinner rapidly and efficiently yourself. You can get over the problem, at least partly, by letting him have his own spoon while continuing to feed him yourself with another. Every few mouthfuls you can reward his own efforts by guiding his own spoon to his mouth. Most babies will be unable to keep the bowl of the spoon uppermost and will turn the spoon over on the way to their mouths which will, of course, deposit most of the spoonful down their fronts. So do invest in a 'pelican' bib. This can save the vast majority of the mess in these early months. Feeding plates with a suction pad on the bottom, to prevent them being removed from high chair or table, will prevent the whole dinner landing on the floor. If you can feed in the kitchen at this stage it does save the carpet. But if you do discourage these early attempts at self-feeding, your baby will very quickly learn that feeding is a passive art and then will be extremely reluctant, if not downright obstructive, when you do want him to feed himself.

With patience, and not a little luck, your baby will be on three meals a day, with something approaching a pint of milk in one form or another, and fruit drinks between meals, by the end of his first year. Do try and make it a rule that he eats nothing between meals, if you want to have the satisfaction of his eating three good meals in the day. It is quite surprising how one or two biscuits between breakfast and lunch can completely ruin his appetite. And do try and keep his sweet consumption down. With a first baby it is fairly easy to restrict this to the odd chocolate button. As sweets appear in the household, with older children, it can be more difficult, but you would be well advised to keep sweets as an end of the meal treat, rather than a continuous source of snacks. Besides being very bad for the teeth and figure, they will stop your child taking sufficient of the right foods at the right time.

Sleep

A well fed baby will go to sleep contented. And of all the other routines in his life, the sleep routine is the one that will keep him and you happiest, if it is a good one.

Babies do need a great deal of sleep and are so much easier to keep happy and cheerful if they get enough. There are few who need less than twelve hours' sleep at night ie from 7 pm to 7 am and some need even more. During the first year, nearly all babies will need to sleep for a period during the morning and afternoon even if it becomes a very short sleep, particularly in afternoon. Later most children are best on just one sleep during the day which can either be during the morning or immediately after lunch. On the whole, late afternoon sleeps will stop your baby settling down well and quickly at night. Exactly how you organise your day will depend upon your other commitments, but life will be much smoother all round if you stick to a reasonably regular routine.

The night's routine should be fairly rigid. I have always found it easier to bath the baby at night as he is then warm, clean and comfortable for going to bed. A warm bath and a warm drink combine to form a powerful sleep inducement. Do try to have time to make going to bed leisurely and good fun. If you just thrust him into bed with a huge sigh of relief that the day is over, he will not settle so peacefully. You may well feel like this, but do not communicate it to him! So make time for a cuddle and a little play; a set routine such as saying goodnight to favourite toys or drawing the curtains together. There are all sorts of little games you can play to make a happy bedtime routine which your babe will learn to recognise as the definite signs of going to

152

bed at night. Later on, of course, looking at a book together, and then the bedtime story, make an easy end to the day. I must repeat from experience, that hurrying the bedtime routine, or trying to take short cuts, never pays off. And, however tired you feel, when bathtime seems just another chore to endure, do stick to it. You will really benefit with long uninterrupted nights' sleep. Up to nine months, or even to the end of the baby's first year, he will often still need a late night drink and this, combined with a nappy change, will often ensure that you can stay in bed until a reasonable hour in the morning. Having successfully weaned your baby onto three main meals in the day, I have found that, by delaying the night feed to 11 pm or so the baby will then often sleep a good eight hours round, to 7 am or even eight in the morning. But, I am afraid, some babies continue to wake a lot earlier than that in the morning and there is then little point in continuing to stay up late. There is absolutely no general rule as to when a baby will drop his late night feed. Some mothers are lucky and, even as early as four or five months, their babies will sleep through. But many continue to need a late night drink most of the way through their first year. Indeed, for some fathers, it is the only feed in which they can completely participate. So I think that you can afford to be flexible about this. However, I do repeat that the one routine to get firmly established, is the bath and bedtime one.

As your baby gets to the end of the first year he will usually be much better on one long sleep during the day than on two short ones. This can be during the morning so that you can get through your household chores with fewer interruptions. Or, if he seems very reluctant to go to bed again in the morning, he may prefer an early lunchtime and then a midday sleep. This can be a marvellous boon to you, because, although the household chores will take longer with him to help, you will have two hours completely free to do something other than housework. I am quite sure that babies and toddlers benefit from a daytime sleep right through their second year and many well into their third year. Do not be in a hurry to wean them off this sleep. A baby can be impossible to amuse towards the end of the day if he is beginning to get very overtired.

Of course, mothers with older children will often have to organise their day around school and playschool trips, but it should be perfectly possible to arrange things so that the day is well organised for everybody.

In the early months a baby will usually accept the darkness quite happily. But, as he gets older, he will often be happier with some light. A landing light left on with the door ajar is often sufficient. Some mothers prefer small night lights left on in the baby's room, but these can be a worry and do sometimes cast shadows which can be disturbing. During the second year your baby will begin to dream and he may well require a sip of drink or just a turn over to get him off to sleep again. And, as he begins to know when he is wet, he might wake as he wets his nappy at night. Lift him then and change him and put him straight back into his cot. You will often be able to do this without waking him completely. Never make the mistake of taking him into your own bed except in very exceptional circumstances, for instance if he is ill. It is much better to stay with him in his own room than to take him into your bed. I have slept in a bed next to the cot with a reassuring hand in the cot, if the babe is ill. This is much preferable to allowing him to think that if he is restless at night he can come into your bed. I am quite sure that this is a mistake and can only lead to a great deal of trouble to abolish the habit. Your bed should be for you and your husband and for no-one else. Of course a romp for all the family is tremendous fun in your bed in the mornings if you can bear it! This I would heartily encourage, but not at night.

Exercise

From a very early age your baby will need regular and vigorous

154

exercise, although the period of time for this is very short at first. Babies love to exercise without a nappy on if you can manage it. Of course this can be much easier in the summer than in the winter. However, during the first six months, let him have a nappy-free kicking time in the pram or on the floor. You can lay him on a sheet, covering a plastic sheet, quiet safely on the carpet. The hammock chair described earlier is a marvellous means of exercise from about three months onwards. The baby can actively kick and bounce himself while watching what you are doing. Do try and encourage him to have an exercise time on his stomach. Some babies do definitely object to this and there is no point in pursuing it if they always cry bitterly. But, just for a short time, with an interesting rattle in front of him, it is invaluable in making him lift his head and will strengthen his back.

Once your baby has started to crawl or squirm along the floor, he will be so actively exercising himself that he will need little encouragement. In fact, you are more likely, at this stage, to be actively trying to discourage him from exploring too far! He will be in everything and exploring everywhere. While your back is turned for only a few minutes he will be across the floor and into your coal bucket. Be wise and reorganise your furniture and best ornaments. Try and make one room baby-proof as far as you can. And always surround him with enough interesting toys and objects to keep him amused within a reasonably prescribed area.

As he progresses, he will try to stand up. You do not have to do anything to encourage this except put an armchair or sofa at the right height within reach, with a favourite toy on it. At this active stage in exploration, a playpen will be invaluable. I must admit to not liking children put in playpens for a prolonged period of time. But I have always used them during this six-month period from crawling to walking proper, for short periods, when you have to be walking in and out. Your attention cannot always be fully on your baby. When the front door bell goes, do not leave him while you go and answer it, unless you put him into his playpen. At least you will know that he is safe, even if he does howl with frustration.

Because the time of usefulness of the playpen is, in my opinion, very short, it can be a great saving if you can borrow rather than buy. And it is worth saying here a little about the different types of playpen. There is the old fashioned one with widely spaced wooden uprights and no floor. If your babe is small, and the space between the uprights too wide, it is possible for him to get part of himself stuck. On the other hand, these upright bars are a great encouragement to standing. The type of playpen in most common use now, is the fishnet one, with a raised and padded floor. Some of the netting in these is so fine a mesh that not only can the baby not get a grasp on it, but the sheer frustration of just trying to look out can be most upsetting. So do choose webbing with a wide mesh, at least an inch across. This will encourage him to stand, will be safe and will not prevent his looking out. If you have any doubts about how the world looks from inside one of these playpens, get inside and check for yourself before you buy.

Once your baby is crawling actively, he will need the increased scope of the room to move about in. He will love to be outside exploring, although I am afraid your washing load will again temporarily increase. Even if the weather is not good, do try and make sure that he does get outside for some part of every day. Children are so much better if they can have even just half an hour outside.

Even when your babe has become a toddler this need for outside activity will continue. Toddlers love the freedom of just being able to trot where they wish, but do make sure that you are not too far behind. They are not very steady when they first start off and at this stage a large wheeled toy of some sort is greatly appreciated. But, although he may get his greatest pleasure from his own activity, do not forget that walking is a new act for him and he will get tired. So do not forsake his pushchair. He will still love long walks in it. He can even get out of it and push it himself a little way.

Milestones and Development

There are two distinct ways of trying to assess a baby's development: by watching and measuring his physical development, and by assessing his mental and social achievements. The two, of course, proceed roughly together, but the former is very much easier to measure. Generally speaking, mothers seem to attach more importance to when their babies sit and walk, but it is just as important to develop mentally, socially and emotionally. By the time your baby is three months old he will be smiling readily at those he knows, and beginning to gurgle when you talk to him. He will be able to lift his head clear of the floor when he is lying face down and will be able to hold on to a rattle for a few seconds. He will wave his arms about excitedly and kick vigorously when lying on his back, which he generally prefers. He will watch you intently within a limited range and will turn his head deliberately to follow your movements. He will have begun to recognise the sound of a feed being prepared and to become excited at this. He will scrabble at the floor when placed face down but not be able to make any movements along it. Loud or sudden noises will continue to alarm him and he will be soothed by his mother's voice or by a cuddle from her. But, if really screaming from hunger, nothing will pacify him except the next feed.

By four months he will be able to hold his head upright in the central position for a few minutes, before he gets tired and it sags forwards. You will be able to support him in a sitting position and the upper part of his back will be straight. But the lower spine will still be rounded. He becomes increasingly aware with every passing week, and is now beginning to vocalise in response to your talking to him.

By about five months he will be able to roll over from his

157

front to his back although very rarely the other way. His head and shoulders will be well off the ground when he is lying on his stomach. He will be able to support himself on his forearms and be able to follow your movements by deliberately turning his head.

By the time he is six months he will be able to roll both ways over and may be able to get up on his hands when he is lying face downwards. He will sit with support but most babies cannot sit alone yet. He may pull up to standing if you hold his hands, but for most babies this is the bouncing stage. He will love to bounce when supported around the chest. He will often, by this stage, be able to move across the floor by squirming on his elbows, but few babies can get up into a proper crawling position yet. He will be laughing and chuckling out loud by now. He will be able to hold on to rattles or toys for several minutes. But nearly everything ends up in the same place, his mouth! Most babies go through this everything to mouth stage, and you are fortunate indeed if yours does not. He is intensely active physically, but will also watch and observe everything interesting that he can see. He will turn immediately to the sound of your voice and will protest when you go away. He will hold on to his bottle when feeding. He will find his feet during this stage and will play with them. He is usually still quite happy to be held and played with by other people and you will think how lucky you are to have a sociable baby.

But, between six and nine months, he will suddenly realise that these people are not you and he will suddenly start clinging to you in a most irritating way. With patience, however, he will still go to those that he sees frequently, but do reassure him when he needs it. Between these months he will finally be able to sit for a considerable length of time with a perfectly straight back. At about the same time he will often learn to stand holding on to a support. He will roll actively both ways and will be able to get himself up into the proper crawling position. Not all babies go through a proper crawling stage, however, but, if they are going to, this is prefaced by a rocking movement on all fours. He might continue to do this for several weeks before he finally takes the plunge and moves forwards. This can be intensely frustrating to watch, but, certainly, no amount of encouraging pushing will make him move off any sooner. Even if your baby never learns to crawl conventionally he can cover quite large distances by rolling, and then squirming, along. He will, by now, be picking up and playing with interesting things, passing them actively from one hand to the other and jabbering to himself the whole time. He will enjoy holding his own solid food such as rusks and will be attempting to hold his own spoon. He is comparatively unsociable at this stage, especially towards new people. He has very little idea of playing with other children.

Between nine and twelve months is the active exploratory stage. He will be crawling everywhere. He will be able to pull himself up to reach things, hopefully, placed out of his reach. He will be able to balance quite well while standing, but will have to bump himself back down again. He will step sideways holding on to the furniture and may let go for a few seconds. This is usually by mistake at first and will usually result in his falling over. He will be developing infuriating habits such as dropping everything onto the floor from his highchair. Giving this its medical name of 'casting', and even recognising that it is a stage that all babies go through, will not help you to curb your irritation, I expect. But, hopefully, he will stop putting everything in his mouth, although you should not rely on this yet. During this stage he will learn the earliest simple games such as 'clap hands' or 'pat-a-cake', 'peep-bo', and may even progress on to waving 'bye-bye' on request. But, rest assured, that yours is not the only baby who will steadfastly refuse to do his 'party-tricks' when asked to do so for an admiring audience. He will play happily on his own for prolonged periods, but will usually like to have you within sight. Hopefully, he is becoming a little more sociable again and he will often spend a long time handing things to and from anybody who has patience enough to do it.

159

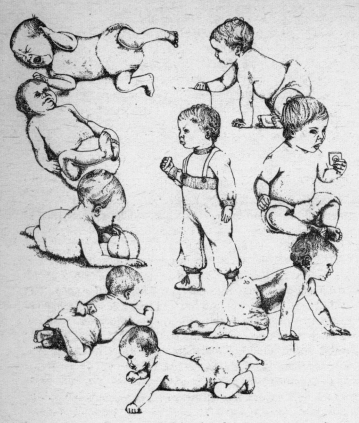

Fig 10 Stages to walking (*see key on opposite page*)

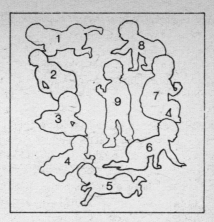

1 6 weeks old—lying still slightly curled. He can lift his head clear but not his shoulders. **2** 3 months old. **3** 5 months old—learning to roll over. Head and shoulders clear of the floor. **4** 6 months old. **5** 7 months —starting to move over the floor. **6** 9 months—crawling actively. **7** 7–9 months—sitting upright with a completely straight back. **8** 9–12 months—pulling to standing. **9** 12–15 months—beginning to walk

He will have started to feed himself at this stage, although he will not be able to prevent the spoon turning over and consequently making a terrible mess. He understands much of what you say at this stage and will bring you things on request. He will shut the door, sit down, or hand things to you if you ask him. If you make a definite point of teaching him any particular words at this stage, do teach him the meaning of the word 'no'. Now that he is mobile, electric plugs, fires and other dangerous objects have a fatal fascination. You cannot go on saying 'no' all the time, so my policy is to concentrate on one particular hazard. With both my children the first delight has seemed to be to pull plugs out of their sockets, and this has been the first thing to earn the occasional smack. You must not keep on and on smacking and remonstrating, so try and remove dangerous objects as much as possible, leaving perhaps one or two that have to be learnt. If you smack more than very occasionally it will have absolutely no effect when you do so. And if you do smack him then make sure that you have explained first and that he has understood. This may sound far fetched at a year but it is really not. It is well worth establishing that when you say 'no' you mean 'no', and if he deliberately does whatever it is again, then he will get a smack.

Somehow it all sounds so easy when you write it down, but it can be most frustrating and irritating and terribly wearing. I think it is the most time-consuming part of child rearing. You will sound like a gramophone record endlessly repeating the same thing. You will have to exercise enormous tolerance so that you do not hit out or shout from sheer exasperation. You will often be exhausted by the end of the day. But if you lose these early battles, then you have lost them for ever. It is no good allowing your toddler total freedom and then expecting him to conform to discipline at school or in adult life. You must not allow a toddler to rule the roost but you will require enormous patience at this early stage. However, there is no need for every day to be a constant round of discipline and criticism. Do put things out of reach that he is not allowed to touch. Allow him to learn reasonably slowly. You cannot smack him for getting into the coal bucket if you leave it in the middle of the floor while you answer the telephone. So make his play area safe and then teach him slowly and systematically.

This active stage of exploration will, of course, continue after his first birthday as, at sometime after this, he will begin to walk. Most babies are walking, albeit unsteadily, by the time they are fifteen months, but this is by no means a rule. Some continue to want a guiding hand well after this. And walking itself is not the summit of achievement. But, generally at about fourteen months, they will take those first few faltering steps unaided across the floor towards you. Your baby will be able to get to his feet alone and let himself down again albeit often still with a bump. He will be rapidly relegated to the floor again if he bumps

162

into anything or if anyone gets in his way. But the energy and application that he will devote to this new skill could well be copied by us when we are trying to acquire a new skill. He will constantly get up again and try again. He will begin to learn new arts such as building bricks. He will begin to enjoy books and, particularly if he has an older brother or sister, he will enjoy scribbling. He will gabble nonstop and will shout to attract attention. He will point at things that he wants and will be able to obey simple instructions. He will understand an enormous amount of what you say to him. He will drink by himself and become much more adept at using a spoon. He will no longer be taking everything to his mouth and he will be playing more constructively with toys. He will also be more constructive when you are trying to dress and undress him and will assist quite actively with sleeves and shoes.

At this stage stairs become a problem and, although he can crawl quite fast upstairs, he may be very slow in learning to come down backwards. Persevere, however, because it is the only way you will achieve peace of mind.

By the time he is eighteen months, your baby is a real toddler. He will prefer to walk most of the time, although he will go back to crawling temporarily if he has another baby to copy. He can usually walk quite safely holding on to something and will love to push and pull wheeled toys around. He may begin to run although he is unable to stop and he will do so by collapsing into a chair. He will climb up and down, on and off chairs and will prefer to try to walk upstairs rather than crawl. He can bend down and retrieve something from the floor without falling over and will get up and down from the floor freely without falling or bumping. He should be able to feed himself quite skilfully with a spoon, although food will continue to be pushed off the plate in an effort to get it onto the spoon. He will have become much more sociable again, loving to play with other children, but tempers will still fly if he tries to remove another child's toy. He has no idea of sharing yet. He will begin to know his own hair, eyes, nose, toes, or other parts of the body and will continually point at interesting things. He will have learnt a variety of different tricks which you will have tremendous fun showing to a good audience. He will begin to love the colours in picture books and may begin to recognise specific objects in them. He is constantly on the move and is in every cupboard that he can find. He will, at this stage, show a remarkable interest in music. He will move rhythmically to the music, try to join in simple nursery rhymes such as 'ring-a-ring-o'-roses' and even attempt to sing. He will be showing a definite preference for using one hand rather than the other. Earlier apparent preference for one hand is generally not significant. Do not try and alter his later preference.

He is constantly demanding during the second half of this second year and can be very exhausting. He will follow you everywhere, wanting to copy what you are doing. He will be never happier than when he is allowed to help. He will be, by the end of his second year, a little boy or girl rather than just a toddler. He will be fully mobile, able to go up and down stairs, and physically very independent. He will help a great deal with dressing and undressing, being able to do the simpler clothes by himself. He will able to run and to throw a ball and will be able to give a fair imitation of a footballer. If it is Christmas he will adore all the unwrapping. He will immediately recognise those people he sees often and will be delighted to see them. He will be able to scribble round and round as well as up and down and will join in any game that you have the energy to play with him.

During the second half of this year he will develop temper tantrums if he is going to. But you should be able to divert his attention and this is usually the best way to deal with it. Do not try to have a confrontation, because you will surely lose. He will love to have other children around, but will still not play with them, preferring to remain independent. Your peace will be further shattered as he learns to open and close doors, turn handles and get into cupboards that you have previously thought safe.

He will be feeding himself and indicating his likes and dislikes at the table. I have deliberately left out the development of speech and the aquiring of the 'potty habit' as these are discussed separately in a later section.

The above section gives a general picture and guide to development.

Variations in Development

I have deliberately not set out a timetable of achievements as not only is this very misleading but it can be very worrying as well. At any stage, if you think that your baby is not progressing at a steady rate, you would be well advised to ask your doctor to check him over, but there are wide variations of the normal rate of development which do not necessarily bear any relationship to subsequent intelligence.

It is possible that the earliness of the first smile and the development of communication is indicative of later intelligence, but even on these one cannot be dogmatic. Certainly physical development, provided that it is fairly steady, bears no relationship whatsoever to future intelligence. And a child of average intelligence with a good stimulating family environment may do infinitely better than a child with slightly better intelligence but a poor background.

Of course the development of the physical, mental, and social skills are of vital importance and overriding interest. They are the way that you will measure your baby's progress, and to have a rough idea of when they normally occur is of great value. But, on the whole, the steadiness of the development of these skills is more important than how quickly they develop. The sequence of lying, propping up on the arms, then standing or walking is the progress that you should watch. There are misleading targets given for an individual achievement that can be as worrying as they are wrong. One of the commonest of these is to say that most children sit up by the time they are six months. Most children can in fact be propped up by the time that they are six months but the true sitting position with a completely straight back is usually not achieved until two or three months after that. Similarly, to quote that most children are walking round about a year is inaccurate. Most children will push to standing by this time. Some will be sidestepping round the furniture but there is often a tremendous gap between this achievement and those first few entirely solo steps. And, indeed, some children will walk quite well while continuing to need a guiding hand by fifteen months, but lack the confidence to step out entirely alone. It is a fact that overweight babies tend to get to their feet more slowly than slimmer ones but this is probably a good thing as they will have to carry excess weight when they do start walking. So, provided that your child progresses, and provided that there are no physical disabilities which are readily checked by your clinic or family doctor, there is far less to worry about than most mothers find. Crawling is a very variable skill and indeed many babies simply do not go through the stage at all. Nearly all manage to progress along the floor before they can walk. But they may squirm along or even shuffle along on their bottoms. If they are going to crawl conventionally, this usually occurs between eight and twelve months, but it is by no means a vital stage. Sometimes a baby is kept more easily amused if he is able to crawl, because he can reach toys and can explore, whereas those who remain static for longer can get frustrated. These babes will require greater ingenuity on your part to keep them amused.

As far as mental development goes, this should also proceed steadily. Your baby will first become aware of you and his immediate surroundings. Then, gradually, he will become aware of, and interested in, things outside his immediate sphere of vision. His participation in activities such as feeding will gradually increase until he can manage all by himself. His enjoyment of organised play, of games and of music will gradually increase. As he learns to play with bricks, for instance, it will be sufficient at first to be able to hold one in his hands, to examine it and perhaps put it into something. Then he will learn to knock the bricks together to make a satisfying noise. Then he will learn to build a modest castle which he will have even greater fun with by knocking it down again. Then he will build more complicated castles and begin to have more sophisticated games with them. And, finally, his games will become filled with make believe, the bricks becoming buildings, bridges and roads and his manipulation of them very complicated. This development of play does seem to follow slightly different patterns in boys and girls. On the whole boys are more physical and direct in their play whereas girls often seem to be more considered. You should encourage your developing child by continually giving him the opportunity to enlarge upon these inventive games. Surprisingly early on, a baby will enjoy looking at a large picture book with good illustrations on everyday objects. He will soon recognise individual pictures and will pat favourite ones vigorously. It does not necessarily require a vast number of toys, but rather a few good ones used with a little ingenuity to stop a child becoming frustrated as he experiments.

Socially a baby has to learn to develop too. He goes through definite stages at remarkably constant times. At no time do I think that it is worthwhile forcing the issue with a child who is upset at a certain social situation. But there are ways of presenting something, and the right approach, together with a tremendous amount of active encouragement, can overcome a very natural resistance to extending the social circle. When your baby is first born, the first few weeks should be spent getting to know you thoroughly. At this time he will usually resent much different handling, unless he is hungry and waiting for food when generally the provider of that food will be acceptable whoever it is. From about three to nine months, most babies are fairly sociable. They love having other children in the house with constant activity going on around them. They love being nursed by those who will play 'peep-bo' or 'round-and-round-the-garden' continuously with them. But, at about the nine or ten month stage, they seem to become clinging again, as though they have just realised that the world is a large place and perhaps it is safer to stick to the known world of 'mum'. Do try not to become too irritated when this stage is reached. Try to encourage him to play with those people who at least are fairly familiar, but do not force the issue with strangers if you can help it. They will emerge from this phase quite satisfactorily, although when faced with complete strangers will continue to need some reassurance. When you go into a room full of people that are strange to your baby—and do not forget that their memories are considerably shorter than yours—do not dump him in the middle of the floor and expect him to start playing, or, even worse, to start performing. Let him sit safely on your lap at first. He will gradually venture away from you when he no longer feels threatened. So try to find something that will interest and divert him if he appears unsure, but do not ever force him. By the time that he has become a proper little toddler, he will mostly have outgrown this extreme shyness, but he will need fairly regular socialising to get him used to accepting other people. I am sure it is worthwhile encouraging your child to be outgoing at this stage. But, of course, there are children who are inherently much less sociable than others and, indeed, social awareness itself develops at vastly different rates in different children. So, again, do not worry if your child cannot be left like other children. Encourage him in a small way to be independent of you and let time enlarge and broaden that independence.

Speech

I have deliberately left speech as a separate developmental section partly because it is so important, and partly because it is even less easy to generalise in the stages of its development. Implicit in the development of speech is the child's ability to hear accurately and any discussion on speech must include a reference to hearing.

From the first month onwards, your baby will be startled by noises and will gurgle when content or excited. A deaf baby will also gurgle like this but will not be startled by a sudden noise.

By the time he is three months old, although he will still cry if startled by a loud noise, you will be able to quieten him by your presence and he will smile and 'coo' at you when you have succeeded in comforting him. Indeed even at this very early stage he will make answering gurgles and coos when spoken to. A deaf baby will communicate when you are directly in his view but he may be considerably startled if you appear suddenly by his cot or pram.

By the time he is six months old he is multi-vocal in that he makes several different single-syllable sounds. He can for instance, make a 'gna' sound, a 'da', 'ma', and 'ga' sound. It is these early sounds, of which 'da' is most commonly the earliest, that give rise to the common myth that 'daddy' is the first word that a baby says. Your baby will, by this time, also be able to gurgle and laugh out loud. The hearing test commonly employed at this time is a set variety of different sounds. These standard sounds are produced briefly behind the baby on each side while his attention is directed forwards by an interesting, but silent, toy. The sounds used are the whispered voice, a soft rattle, a cup rattling gently against a spoon, rustling paper, and a bell. Most babies are remarkably co-operative but the response to the sounds at this age is not immediate. The baby seems to take a while to catch on.

By the time the child is nine months, provided that his hearing is good, he will be vocalising deliberately to attract attention. He will shout or call, listen for an answer and then shout again. He will babble continuously, using repeated consonant sounds such as 'da-da-da-', 'ma-ma-ma', and 'ba- ba- ba'. He will be trying to imitate adult sounds that are interesting. such as 'brmm-brmm' or smacking lips or coughs. He will be understanding 'bye-bye' and will often wave on request, or say the words, but he will usually fail to do both together! He will be able to clap hands and play 'peep-bo'. He can begin to understand quite a variety of the common commands. He will understand 'come on', 'let's feed the dog', 'let's shut the door'. His understanding will greatly exceed his ability to verbalise.

By the time he is a twelve to fourteen month old, he may well be able to speak a few simple, but recognisable, words. These will be very inaccurate and may only be understood by his family. However, if the sounds that he makes are constant for a given question or object, they may be interpreted as meaningful speech. One of the earliest sounds that can be learnt rewardingly are animal noises, especially if you can demonstrate the animal regularly to remind him. Dogs and cats are readily visible to nearly every child in the country, so that 'miaow' and 'woof-woof' form an early part of many children's vocabulary. But, apart from the actual words, which come slowly, he will have an enormous range of sounds that he will jabber continuously and often tunefully. Again, at this stage, his understanding is very much greater than his ability to communicate. His methods of asking will usually be an urgent torrent of babbled sounds. But if you ask him to point out 'the light', 'the dog', 'daddy', etc, he will do so readily. He will immediately respond and turn to his own name and will carry out simple commands such as 'shut the door' and 'pass me your shoes'. His response to the hearing tests given above are by now immediate, provided that he is not distracted by something more interesting than the test sounds.

By the time he is eighteen months old, he has a definite range of recognisable noises. I say 'noises' because often the words are so inaccurate that they are still only instantly appreciated by the family or close aquaintances. Also, they tend to be used only in the familiar surroundings of home. It is often a source of irritation that your baby will not perform to command. He is certainly understanding the means of communication by this time, even if he cannot accurately reproduce it. He will point to a known object and then smile contentedly when you produce the right word. He points to anything that interests him. He continues to talk to himself constantly and will join in communal activities such as 'ring-a-ring-o'-roses'. He begins to know the parts of his body and will point them out on request.

By the time he is two he has an increased range of words which are much more readily recognisable by other people. He generally knows his own name to say. He goes on chattering to himself echoing the same word or phrase continuously. He will be constantly demanding to know the name of objects that interest him.

It is during the third year that the biggest, or rather the most obvious, advance in speech is made. The child learns to put two or more words together to form small sentences. Instead of just using nouns, he learns to use adjectives and verbs. He will start using the pronouns 'I' and 'you', instead of always referring to people by name. During this year he will learn to ask 'why' and the addition of this word to his vocabulary will successfully abolish any peace that you had before! This is the commonest time for stuttering to develop as he struggles to put into words thoughts that occur quicker than he can translate them. If he does start to stutter never make an issue out of it. Help him out by giving him a few of the more difficult leads. Slow him down by distracting him and joining in the conversation to give him pause, rather than correcting him. Once the initial flood of eagerness that caused the stuttering has subsided, he will start again perfectly well. He will be joining in simple nursery rhymes by now even if it is only the ends of every line or indeed just the punch line.

The time scale that I have given here is very approximate. I have not said that a child will be speaking so many words by a certain age, as this seems to me just to worry mothers unduly. More than anything else, the development in speech varies enormously from child to child. It is commonly accepted that, whereas boys are more physical earlier, girls tend to speak earlier. I see no reason to contradict this. There is no doubt that some children miss out some of the stages of speech learning, or at least these are not recognisable. From simple monosyllabic utterances they will suddenly, after an apparently very prolonged period of time, start speaking in whole sentences or phrases. Some people maintain that second children speak quicker than first because they copy their older siblings. Others are equally sure that second children speak slower, because their older siblings understand their needs without their having to ask specifically. I think it is much less a result of their position in the family than a child's individual variation.

I believe that you can definitely speed up the progress of speech learning once it has started, but you cannot fundamentally alter the rate at which he will be able to imitate. Once he has learnt to copy the individual sounds, you will be able to teach him new words very quickly, if you do so with perseverance and patience. For this reason, many first children may speak more accurately more quickly, simply because we spend more time actively talking 'at' them. If, for instance, you say 'light' every time you turn one on, your child will tend to learn it more quickly than if you call out in an aside to an older child, 'turn the light on will you'; the child will quickly understand the pattern of the speech enough to obey without being able to reproduce the component parts of the speech.

But while I feel it is very important to speak in a manner which will teach, I see no sense in introducing baby-talk, for example, introducing an animal as a 'gee-gee', only to change it later to 'horse'. I believe a child will learn to say 'dog' just as quickly as he will learn to say 'doggy-woggy'! Not, of course, that a child will not introduce his own way of making things easier to say. He will adapt difficult words without our help and his, at least, will be an adaptation of the word that he will ultimately have to learn. As in all aspects of the management and

172

teaching of children, consistency is of the utmost importance. So do try not to let your pet be a 'pussy' one day, a 'miaow-miaow' the next and a 'cat' on the third. But, by all means, say that the cat says 'miaow-miaow'. He may well enjoy the sound that the cat says more than the name itself. But try and make your teaching sensible and consistent.

And, above all, as I so constantly repeat, do not worry if your child's speech seems to be developing more slowly than that of your next-door neighbour's child. Provided that his hearing has been checked and passed, and provided that he starts to 'phonate' and then to copy, however inaccurately, his speech will develop. And do not, at an early stage, correct all his infantile forms of speech. They will come right later and you may well avoid the stuttering stage.

Nappy Routine and Potty Training

Nappies and their washing can take up an inordinate amount of time unless you establish a good routine. In this, of course, we are vastly better off today with the appearance of the chemical soaking solutions. They do vary a lot and I have no doubt myself that Napisan is the most effective. Your solution should be made up fresh, in a bucket with a lid, every morning (or evening) according to your own household routine. I keep the bucket well out of the way of flying toddlers in a safe corner of the bathroom, but anywhere handy is fine so long as it is out of the way. Wet nappies can just be dropped straight in but I rinse them first under the tap, simply because that way you can get more nappies clean in one solution. Dirty nappies should be rinsed of all solid matter before going into the solution. Probably the simplest way of doing this is to flush them down the toilet, making sure that you keep a firm hold on one corner. The average size bucket can hold six or seven nappies and cleanse them properly and this is usually sufficient for one day. It is probably true that if you then rinse the nappies thoroughly the next day, that is all the washing required. But the difficulty I always find, is rinsing them adequately.

If you are lucky enough to have an automatic washing machine I feel that they are far better put through a minimum wash and full rinse routine in addition to the soaking in Napisan. If you are among the many who use the launderette then again they can go through with your white wash, having already been cleansed and disinfected in the solution. If you have an ordinary washing machine, or twintub, then, again, put them through with the whites. If you wash by hand, then, although it is a chore to do so, I still think it is safer to wash them as well, as if they are soaped then you can be sure when all the soap is out. And nappies do require a lot of rinsing. The reason that it is worthwhile being so particular about the rinsing of your nappies is that any chemical or soap left in them is a potent aggravator of nappy rash, and you do want to avoid that at all costs. Washing the nappies need not be a great chore if you deal with them immediately, rather than leaving them for an hour or so when you mistakenly think you will have more time.

With a young baby you can be sure that the vast majority of his dirty nappies will occur just after a feed and so a regular change after every four-hourly feed will keep him reasonably clean and dry all day.

As your baby gets older and the periods of play lengthen, then you should definitely change him before putting him down for a rest as well as after every meal.

Many people use a thin muslin nappy inside a towelling one and some use nappy liners as well. Indeed, I think that these probably do have advantages, but it is of far more importance to change him regularly than what type of nappies you use. Provided that towelling nappies are well washed and well rinsed, they will remain soft and I have never used muslin nappies or nappy liners.

As your baby gets older you will have to decide on your method of potty or toilet training. It is best to examine the facts first. By the time your baby is a year old, and often before, he will be conscious of, and uncomfortable in, a dirty nappy. But, of course, he will be unable to do anything about preventing it. Soon after a year he will be able to indicate when he has soiled his nappy, and by fifteen months he will often indicate when he is wet. The commonest and greatest stimulus to a bowel action is food. This is called the gastro-colic reflex. If your child has a good meal, within ten minutes or so he will feel the need to have his bowels open. This will not happen at every meal, but it will be quite apparent to many mothers that there is a pattern to his habits. He recognises the need to pass water much later on and, indeed, does so only at the last minute. With these facts in our possession, I would recommend the following pattern of potty training. But, while I am quite convinced this is the best, it is also of extreme importance that you do not see the task as a battle between your babe and yourself and that failure and accidents do not worry you. Your attitude to the training will certainly influence the ease with which you achieve the desired aim.

I would start sitting your baby on a comfortable potty for a few minutes after meals (the three main ones) from about nine months. He is able to sit firmly by this time and, if the pot is comfortable, he will play with a favourite toy quite happily for a minute or so. He is usually unable to stand alone at this time and so the temptation to do so will be removed. Because he is so young, you will not expect a result, so it will be a tremendous bonus and one less nappy if you do manage to catch his one main bowel movement of the day. You will be establishing a routine of sitting on the potty after meals, so that when it does become important he is already used to what is expected. Your baby will not like sitting on an ice-cold potty, nor on one that is either too big or too small. And he will not like being plonked on the floor with nothing to do. So make it worth his while to sit there for a moment or two. Reserve a favourite toy or even look at a book with him while he is there. And do not leave him sitting

175

there for hours. It is not worth it, he will resent it, become bored and finally reject the idea altogether.

By the time he is a year you will be 'catching' the majority of his motions and, if you are anything like me, you will welcome the lightening of your washing load. He will, therefore, be being kept much cleaner and more comfortable and will begin to resent having wet pants too. It is worthwhile, now, offering the potty at extra times, such as after his daytime rest. If you show enough enthusiasm every time that you succeed, and fail to show your irritation when you do not, then he will be delighted with his own performance. He will recognise it as all his own work and will want to show any willing audience.

By the time that he is eighteen months he will usually have achieved bowel control and be able to give you sufficient warning as to when it is about to occur.

By the time he is two years, with regular potting, he will be dry during the day and indeed you may achieve this well before his second birthday. But, because you are doing all this gradually and saving washing and nappy rash at the same time, you will not need to get uptight or neurotic about it and will accept success almost without noticing it. When I say 'regular potting' I do not mean that you should follow your child about with the pot every five minutes. A reasonable timetable would be; after breakfast, before and after his morning nap, after lunch, once during the afternoon, again after tea and, finally, before bed if there is a reasonable gap between tea and this time.

If you have introduced the potty in this unhurried, unfussed way, with no sense of frustration, simply because when you start you will not be expecting any success, you will not create any resentment or difficulty in your child. I am quite sure that resentment creeps in if you attempt to force the issue at a slightly later date, confronting him with the pot and your high expectations all at once. Do not ever confront him with the feeling of 'perform or else'. He will not and the positions of the inevitable fight will be taken up.

176

Now, while I believe that this is easily the most sensible and painfree method of potty training, I do accept that other routines have worked well. It would be reasonable, when considering the facts, to only offer the pot when it means something, that is at about fifteen months. But by this time your child will be toddling and his first impulse on being sat where he does not want to be sat will be to get up and walk away. So if you do choose this way do make sure that the floor round the potty is liberally strewn with favourite toys. Now, there is another method by which you do not offer the potty until the child is old enough to know what is expected of it, that is after two years. I have known this to work apparently miraculously in that, from being completely untrained, the child is trained within a fortnight. This method certainly reduces any tension that might creep in by my method, but does absolutely nothing for the skin of your child's bottom and perineum while he is untrained. The urine volume increases and the motion becomes steadily more adult and unpleasant as the child grows and I feel this must be most un-unpleasant for the child, while being the most awful chore for the mother. However, if this works for you and your temperament, then I cannot really condemn it. But, if you are open to suggestion, then I would strongly recommend that a steadier and earlier approach is preferable.

Girls, of course, continue to sit down to pass water and have their bowels open when they progress to the adult toilet. And here, do get an adaption for the toilet seat to make it smaller. No child will go readily if they are struggling to stop falling down the pan. But, at some point, you must encourage boys to pass water standing up. By all means show him what is expected of him by letting him go to the toilet with daddy, providing that daddy is willing. But also try and find some time in the day when you can be fairly sure of catching him actually passing water. I have found, for instance, immediately on standing up in the bath my son invariably passed water! Make capital out of this frustrating habit and catch it. He will be thrilled and learning will be fun. And when your son does graduate to standing up at the toilet, give him a solid base to stand up on—an upturned box or a small stool. He will then be able to have great fun going along on his own.

Getting your child dry at night can take a considerable time after he has achieved dryness by day. So, having achieved the latter, relax and wait before trying to get him to go through the night as well.

By the time your child is two and a half, if he needs lifting at night, it is worthwhile arranging to do this just before you go to bed. That way he will probably be dry until 11 pm or so, and then might well go through until the next morning dry. I do not necessarily think it is worth waking your child if he does not naturally wake once during the night anyway. That way you can distress him by waking him and he is unlikely to pass water while distressed. Having said this, however, I must admit that I have always tried lifting as a means of getting through the night. But, if he does not wake naturally, and is resentful at being woken, then if you leave it until he is nearer three, you will often succeed quite naturally. The only other reason for which you might be well advised to establish a lifting routine, is if he soaks the bed at night. There is no hard and fast rule as to when you can get your baby dry at night, but there are things you can do to help. It is really not wise to let him drink copiously just before going to bed. Talk to your child about it and tell him how grown up it will be for him to succeed. But do be careful not to make an issue out of it. Sometimes the very fact that he continues to wear nappies can continue the habit of night wetting. I must say that I have been caught out that way myself. So when you have a comparatively free week, talk to him about it and say that now is the time to stop night nappies. It can work just like that, but I would not try this until he is about three.

There is nothing you should worry about physically, unless your child achieves dryness at night and then suddenly relapses. If, for instance, he has been dry at night for several months and then starts wetting again, then there could be something physically wrong, such as a water infection, and you would be wise to check with your doctor.

This whole question of training is difficult not, I think, because of any inherent difficulty, but because of the emotions and hang-ups that have become associated with it. If you can abolish your own anxieties and tension about the subject, you will be at least half way there. Your baby's natural development will go a further way towards it. And a little bit of routine will finally clinch the matter. You might then be able to enjoy even this aspect of your child's development.

Teething

Your baby will grow twenty milk teeth, ten in the upper jaw and ten in the lower. The first to appear are usually the lower central incisors. These can appear any time after six months and usually before ten months. The upper central and lateral incisors follow rapidly and are usually present by the end of the first year. The lower lateral incisors are the next to appear and may come any time during the first half of the second year. The first molars appear at roughly the same time. The canines appear next and are usually present by the end of the second year. The second molars are the last to appear and may arrive any time from twenty months to two and a half years.

Even given these approximate dates, the time of eruption does vary greatly. In my opinion a baby who is weaned early will, on the whole, gain his teeth earlier than a baby who is entirely breast-fed for a prolonged period. Maybe this is just as well, as the appearance of the teeth can summarily halt the breast-feeding! When the teeth do erupt they can come suddenly and several may erupt together. You will know when they are about to come because the tops of the gums flatten out and a thin grey line appears along the gum as the tooth can be seen just below the surface.

179

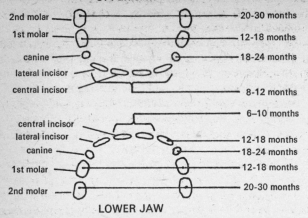

2nd molar	20-30 months
1st molar	12-18 months
canine	18-24 months
lateral incisor	
central incisor	8-12 months
	6–10 months
central incisor	
lateral incisor	12-18 months
canine	18-24 months
1st molar	12-18 months
2nd molar	20-30 months

LOWER JAW

Fig 11   Approximate time of eruption of teeth

There are more symptoms and ailments attributed to teething than to any other facet of child development. The vast majority of these ailments are wrongly thus attributed and, indeed, it can be very dangerous to attribute certain symptoms to teething without first having a check up with your doctor.

There is no doubt that children can be grizzly when the teeth are actually erupting, but this only continues for a few days at the most. They undoubtedly chew on their hands and gums and I think it is probably fair to say that the following symptoms also seem to occur in conjunction with teething more often than not.

1 A slightly higher colour on the cheeks during actual eruption.

2 Slightly odd motions (*not* diarrhoea) for a few days.

3 A few spots around the mouth.

But the only specific physical changes during teething are an increase in salivation and soreness of the gum while the tooth is actually pushing through. As a result of increased salivation and chewing on the gum, babies can develop spots around the mouth simply as a result of chafing against moist skin. It is possible, because of the increased tendency to chew anything, however unsuitable or dirty, the motions can be a little upset. But, more than all this cannot and should not be attributed to teething. And I must point out that it is not necessary to have any symptoms at all. Many babies cut their teeth perfectly well without any fuss.

Teething of itself does not cause diarrhoea and vomiting. It does not cause high temperatures, or febrile convulsions. It does not cause widespread rashes or spots. Indeed, teething has been used as an excuse for all the minor ailments occurring incidentally in childhood. There is no doubt that if a child has an illness while he is also cutting some teeth, then that illness is likely to be made somewhat worse. But if your child is ill, he should be checked by your doctor and his teething not allowed to be the scapegoat for a real infection. Indeed, it can be very dangerous to ignore such symptoms as severe diarrhoea. If your baby has gastroenteritis, the medical name for the infection that causes severe diarrhoea, it is dangerous for him not be treated. And if he has a high temperature, do not assume he is just teething. Make sure that your doctor looks to see if he can find any real infection. Your child should cut his teeth with minimal disruption to his sleep, digestion and food habits. If he wants to chew give him something suitable to chew on. And if he is more than mildly unwell, do see your doctor.

Common Complaints and When to Panic

There are some ailments which are so common as to affect nearly all children at some point during their first year. They deserve individual attention.

1 *Nappy Rash*

I will deal with this only briefly here, as I have mentioned it fairly fully in this and earlier sections. By far the most important thing to re-state is that prevention is so much better than cure. Do not leave your baby wet or dirty for longer than is absolutely necessary. Do wash and rinse your nappies really thoroughly. Do protect the delicate skin of the perineum with a really good greasy cream. Do cleanse the perineal area really thoroughly at each nappy change. Do bathe your babe regularly once a day, or more often if he develops loose stools for any reason. If, in spite of all these precautions, your baby does develop a nappy rash, and they do occur in the best regulated families, then try the following measures.

1   Cleanse the buttock area with lotion such as Johnson's baby lotion at every nappy change.

2   Apply a baby cream liberally to the affected area.

3   Apply vaseline as a protective coat to all the surrounding area.

4   Use an Ever-Dri nappy liner to keep the perineum drier.

5   Leave the buttock naked with no nappy for some time every day.

6   Change the nappies more frequently.

7   Leave the foreskin severely alone in baby boys while the buttocks are sore.

There is no particular virtue in any special creams or lotions. It is time and cleansing, with any cream, that will eventually do the trick. If the nappy rash is persistent, it is possible that your baby has thrush and this can be specifically treated by your doctor. So do check with him if you have any doubts.

2   Coughs and Colds

At some time during his first year your baby is almost certain to have a cold. If he has older brothers and sisters then this cold is liable to come earlier than if the child is a first baby. Whenever he gets it, your baby will become irritable and very snuffly. He will find sucking a bottle, if he is at that stage, very difficult. This will put him off his food, and this, in turn, will make him sleep less soundly. You will, I am afraid, have several troubled days and nights. The acute stage of misery, however, does not last long, but, unfortunately, because of their inability to blow their noses, the after effects of running noses will seem to last much longer than in adults. The younger the baby the more difficult it is to manage.

You will find that a very young baby is more easily managed on smaller, more frequent, feeds at this stage and as soon as he will take a full feed you will know that the worst is over. Your greatest contribution, apart from keeping him well fed, is to endeavour to keep his nose clear particularly just before he is going to bed. Many people advocate cotton buds to keep noses clear, but I feel much happier using the rolled corner of a tissue. This way you can remove the sticky mucus just as well and stand much less chance of pushing solid matter back into the nose. You will also be in no danger of damaging the very soft tissues of the nose. If he is feverish, a small amount of a mixture, such as Calpol, which you can obtain from your doctor, will help to keep him less irritable. If your baby's temperature rises on the second or third day, and he develops a cough, rubs his ear or seems to be in pain, then you should consult your doctor. A cold can so easily be complicated by bronchitis or an ear infection.

You can guard against this spread of infection by keeping him indoors during the initial two or three days of infection. It does no good at all to expose him to cold and wet while he has an active infection. When he has got to the 'just runny nose' stage, and if the weather is favourable, then, in fact, it can help to give him a breath of fresh air. But do not be afraid to cosset him in the first few days, especially if he is very young.

If your babe is fortunate enough not to have a cold until the end of his first year, then it will not be so worrying for you, although it can still cause him to be very irritable. He will often go right off solid food and you would be wise not to push it. Keep him drinking well and let him eat just what he fancies.

Keep him warm but do not smother him in a lot of extra blankets. You can push up his temperature in this way and thus increase his irritability. Do make sure that when your babies or children are ill they get as much sleep as you can possibly manage. This way they reserve all their energies for fighting off the infection.

You cannot shield a child from contact with all other children who have infections, but if you know that an acquaintance has had a bad cold, then it is only sensible to avoid him for a few days, especially in the first few months of your baby's life. Even colds can be very worrying in a very young baby. And, similarly, if your toddler or child has a cold then it is only fair not to let him play with other very young children.

If, at any time during such an infection, you are at all worried about your baby's breathing, then do consult your doctor.

3 *Diarrhoea and Vomiting*

Amongst all the minor ailments that affect so many children in their first year, this is the potentially most dangerous. Tiny babies do lose fluid and become dehydrated very easily and, indeed, can become severely ill very suddenly. Diarrhoea, in the first year of life particularly, can never be taken lightly. But there are many grades of severity of diarrhoea and, in fact, the term is used to cover a very wide variety of different motions.

I do not mean you to panic instantly if your baby passes loose motions in the usual volume and no more frequently than normal. This can mean simply that you have tried a new food, while weaning, that does not agree with him. For instance, too much meat protein too early, or too much of some vegetable, can upset him sufficiently to make his motion much softer than usual for twenty-four or forty-eight hours. If he remains eating normally, and appears well, there is usually little need to worry. Simply go back over the diet of the previous twenty-four hours and exclude anything new. If the motion persists looser than normal, then it is usually wise to revert to a bland diet and half-strength milk for twenty-four hours. If there is still no improvement, then you should consult your doctor.

Next in severity is the twenty-four hour gastric-flu type of diarrhoea that is nearly always accompanied by vomiting. It is useless to keep offering food if your baby is being sick. You should offer fluid drinks only but plenty of them. It is wise to dilute the milk feeds to half strength and, if this is not tolerated, then offer clear fluids such as diluted fruit juice every two hours. It will not harm him to have fluids only for twenty-four hours, provided that he gets enough. As soon as the vomiting has stopped, which it usually does very quickly once food is withdrawn, re-introduce half-strength milk. If this is tolerated for three feeds, increase the strength to three-quarter-strength milk. If this is tolerated for three feeds then re-introduce full-strength milk. Let your baby remain on milk alone for another twenty-four hours, then start cautiously re-introducing solid food again. The basic rules to remember when dealing with this type of infection are, first, to rest the stomach as quickly and completely as possible and, secondly, to get back to a full diet sufficiently slowly. It is useless to start back on a normal diet as soon as the vomiting has ceased. You will surely start it all up again. Many mothers tend to do this in the mistaken impression that the babe must be hungry after being starved for so long. If you recall a a stomach upset in yourself, you will remember that you do not feel hungry again immediately. While these are good guidelines for the management of mild gastro-enteritis, you should not be afraid to get your own doctor's advice early on, if at any time you are worried.

However, if your young baby develops the kind of diarrhoea that is almost like water, and it is present at every nappy change you should consult your doctor immediately. Babies can lose an enormous amount of vital body fluid very quickly with watery diarrhoea, without even vomiting, although this, of course, will aggravate it. In severe diarrhoea, the motion can be so fluid that it may be mistaken for ordinary urine or water. So be on your guard. You will know that your baby has an infection, because he will be listless and off his food. The smaller the baby the more immediate should be your call to your doctor. His treatment will be much as that outlined above, unless he considers the baby should be in hospital. But call him in for his advice sooner, rather than later.

I have so far dealt with the combination of diarrhoea and vomiting that means an actual infection of the digestive system. But there are many conditions in which a baby can vomit without having diarrhoea. In fact, one of the commonest symptoms of any infection in a baby is vomiting, even if the infection has nothing to do with the stomach. For instance, an infection of the middle ear will often start with vomiting and a high temperature. Here, again, if your babe is off his food, with a high temperature, and vomiting, the only wise course is to consult your doctor. All these points are the more immediate, the younger the baby. But, on the whole, a baby who has previously been feeding well and who suddenly vomits a feed, has an infection, until proved otherwise.

The vital rule remains that any child who vomits, or who has diarrhoea, needs a lot of fluid to replace what he is losing although he can easily do without any solid food.

4   Skin Spots and Eczema

This section will deal in general with the skin and its problems and not specifically with the 'spotty diseases' which are dealt with later.

Because the condition of the skin is so obvious to anyone who sees or handles your baby, its health is apparent very quickly and therefore can become important out of all proportion to you. When your babe has spots on his face, as so many do at one time or another, it will be readily apparent and will therefore be a constant anxiety and often an irritation to you.

The commonest of the skin disorders of babyhood is the nappy rash and this has been dealt with already.

Second is the form of skin disorder which results in cradle cap. Again this has been fully dealt with earlier.

The next most common are the widespread pimply spots on reddened skin which constitute a sweat rash. This is extremely common in the first few months of life, particularly on the face and neck. More babies are overclothed than underclothed and, if they become too hot and are lying on a plastic sheet, and even more so if they are wearing, or are covered with, nylon, they very readily develop these sweat spots. From this description, the treatment must be obvious. Do not overclothe the babe; use only cotton sheeting; use a real rubber sheet instead of plastic, and bathe the whole baby once a day.

The skin of a young baby is very sensitive and this type of spots does occur very readily. When a baby dribbles excessively, when he regurgitates a little in his cot, or when, because of teething, he produces a lot more saliva than usual, it takes very little rubbing of his face in this moisture to produce the same type of small spots as in a sweat rash. Again the management must be obvious. Keep some small squares of cotton sheeting which can be continually replaced under the baby's head without having to change the whole bed.

By far the majority of spots and skin problems that appear in the first year of life can be attributed to such ordinary and mundane things as the above. But the question that is always asked, if a skin problem is not readily solved, is 'Is it eczema?' Infantile eczema is a specific skin disease of the face, head and limbs which can occur in the first year of life and which may be associated with asthma in later life. The disease usually begins in the first six months and is rare after a year. It is generally considered to be an allergy, but the cause is very rarely found. There is often a family history of some type of allergy.

The spots begin as little pimples, become blisters and, as such, are intensely irritating. The babe will scratch and they then go on to form crusts. The spots come and go apparently quite haphazardly. Nearly all the cases clear themselves by the second or third year.

The treatment is basically: a) to prevent scratching; b) to prevent sweating which can make it worse, and c) to stop using soap and water on the affected areas. Nearly all children can be treated quite successfully at home. Occasionally, if it becomes very widespread, a time in hospital may be necessary, but this is rare. Your doctor will provide you with a cream which usually has a coal-tar base, and if the babe is unduly restless at night, then he may supply something to help him sleep.

It is always worth while checking his diet for anything which appears to make his eczema worse. Occasionally, some offending factor will become obvious. But this is rare, and it is nearly always a question of patient conservative treatment, and nearly all cases disappear spontaneously. If your babe is unfortunate enough to have infantile eczema then take heart that it will almost certainly go. He will not always have a bad skin. And it is by no means always associated with asthma in later life.

5 Temperatures and Convulsions

Children develop temperatures often and remarkably easily. They also develop high temperatures more rapidly and generally with less significance than adults. In fact some people will maintain that it is positively harmful for mothers to have a thermometer in the house because they will be alarmed so frequently. I do agree with this, but would stress that it is the way the thermometer is used and the interpretation given to the temperature, rather than the temperature itself, that counts. Having said this, however, all temperatures do mean something, although it is always wise to look at the child first and the temperature second! If your child is bouncing around the room happily, albeit flushed, and yet the thermometer tells you that his temperature is 102 degrees, do not panic too soon. He is obviously not as ill as his temperature would suggest.

188

Like any young animal, the brain and nervous system is excitable and, as such, is likely to overact. Because of this, children do quite commonly have convulsions or fits with high temperatures. It is probably how quickly the temperature rises, rather than how high it reaches, that counts. For this reason, even if your child is not too unwell, if his temperature is high, you should make every attempt to reduce it. This means:

1 Not wrapping him up too closely.
2 Not letting him crouch over a fire or stove.
3 Giving him aspirin or an aspirin-containing compound.
4 Giving him plenty of drinks.
5 Finally, if his temperature remains very high, bathing him gently with a flannel dipped in tepid water.

At this point I must reiterate that temperatures and convulsions do not occur as a result of teething. If a child has a temperature for another reason, and he is, incidentally, teething, the teething process can be accelerated. But the temperature and the convulsion, if he should have them, are not due to the teething itself.

All of the common infections, 'the spotty diseases', will produce temperatures, as will most viral infections. A young child with an ordinary cold can produce quite a high temperature. Diarrhoea and vomiting will also produce a temperature. Usually the cause of the temperature will be apparent and it is the symptoms of the disease rather than the temperature itself which will make you call your doctor. The temperature is often just a confirmation that the infection which you suspected is there. And indeed, if the baby or child is unwell with symptoms that worry you, you should call your doctor even if there is no temperature—some virus infections cause very little rise in temperature, even though the baby can be quite ill.

So if your baby has a high temperature and you cannot find the cause, do let your doctor know. And if he is subject to convulsions and has a high temperature, do take the measures mentioned above to reduce the temperature while waiting for the doctor.

If your child does have convulsions with a temperature, they are likely to continue to occur until his third year. A convulsion of this sort is a brief generalised twitching of the whole body which will stop by itself, leaving no residual signs. The important thing to do if your child does have a convulsion, is to turn him onto his side, making sure his tongue is pulled well forward and not dropping backwards to impede his breathing. You should sponge him with tepid water to reduce his temperature. Do not try to restrain him, but if he is clenching his teeth, put a spoon padded with a handkerchief, or a wooden spoon, between his teeth to stop him biting his tongue. And do make sure that your own doctor, and any other doctor who treats him for anything at any time, knows that he is liable to have convulsions with high temperatures. You must also inform the person who does your vaccinations and immunisations for you.

6 'Panic Signs' in the Young Child

It does not help of course to panic at any stage. But I list here a few symptoms that should make you call your doctor straight away.

1 Any difficulties with breathing for any cause, apparent or not.

2 Diarrhoea, with or without vomiting in a very young baby, and the same in a slightly older child, if it does not resolve quickly.

3 A very young baby who suddenly goes off his food and appears listless.

4 A high temperature with an ill child.

5 A convulsion if your baby has never had one before. Even if you have, unfortunately, had to become used to dealing with convulsions, you should let your doctor know every time one occurs.

6   Any illness that is accompanied by a discharge from the ear.

7   A combination of headache, vomiting and temperature.

8   Unconsciousness, for whatever cause.

The Spotty Diseases—Common Infectious Diseases

I give here a brief outline of the common infectious diseases and have prepared a table of the incubation periods of the commonest of these. The days given are approximate. I have detailed the time during which he is infective and, therefore, the time that he should be isolated, as far as possible, from other children. Quarantine, as such, is not often practised now and there is not much evidence that it is of any value except in the rare case of smallpox. Indeed, in the case of rubella (German measles), young girls should be encouraged to get the disease because of the dangers it carries if contracted during pregnancy. Similarly, boys should be encouraged to get mumps before the age of puberty, because of the danger of mumps affecting the testicles.

I have included the little recognised illness known as roseola infantum, because it does occur quite frequently in babyhood and its appearance, and particularly the very high temperature associated with it, can be alarming.

1   *Measles*

This is a very common virus infection which is rare before five months, because the mother passes on her immunity; commonest between four and eight years, because most children catch it at school. Of course, if you have older children already at school, then younger siblings are more likely to get it earlier. It is most common in the winter and spring and is caught by direct contact. It is a very infective disease and is at its most infective before the spots come out.

The illness starts suddenly with a rising temperature in a very

191

DISEASE	INCUBATION PERIOD	YOUR CHILD WILL BE INFECTIVE			HE SHOULD BE ISOLATED FOR
		FROM	TO		
Measles	7–14	6 days before the rash	TO	5 days after temperature becomes normal	1 week after the rash appears
Chicken Pox	7–21 (commonly 14–18)	1 day before the rash	TO	6 days after the appearance of the rash	1 week after the rash appears
Mumps	14–28	2 days before swelling	TO	disappearance of swelling	until swelling gone
German Measles	14–21	1 day before rash	TO	2 days after appearance of rash	until rash gone
Polio	7–21 (commonly 7–14)	3 days before symptoms	TO	unknown—several weeks	3 weeks
Scarlet Fever	1–5	onset of sore throat	TO	clear tests on throat swab	1 week after onset of treatment, or until swabs clear
Whooping Cough	7–14	2 days before symptoms	TO	6 weeks after cough starts	at least 4 weeks after start of cough
Roseola Infantum	7–14 (commonly 10)	NOT VERY INFECTIVE			unnecessary
Smallpox	7–21 Short incubation period in inoculated persons	3 days before rash	TO	*all* scales off of *all* skin healed	until all scabs off and all skin healed
Diphtheria	1–6	onset of symptoms	TO	clear throat swabs	not less than 4 weeks

miserable child. He usually has a running nose and, most commonly, red and discharging eyes. His tongue is furred and his throat red. He will be off his food, the light will trouble him and he often has a dry irritating cough. During the early stage of the illness, little greyish spots, known as Koplik's spots, develop on the inside of the cheek. These are only found in measles. Towards the end of this early phase, the temperature falls and the rash appears. It appears at first as a blotchy red rash behind the ears, and then rapidly spreads to the whole body. The rash starts off pale pink and extremely itchy. The individual little spots then join together and become darker. The whole rash lasts about six days. As the rash appears, the temperature goes up and the child feels ill again. The cough, which was dry, will then often become productive. Finally, as the rash fades, the skin is left stained slightly brown.

The commonest complications of measles are ear infections and lung infections, such as bronchitis and, less commonly, pneumonia. The incidence and dangers of both these complications are much reduced with the use of penicillin. Many children, especially younger ones, are very prone to a form of gastro-enteritis with measles and, very rarely indeed, the disease may be complicated by an encephalitis arising as the rash fades, occasionally accompanied by convulsions.

It is very rare to have measles twice. One attack usually confers complete immunity for life.

2 Chicken Pox

This is another common infectious disease. It is rare under a year and is transmitted by direct contact with infected droplets from the nose and mouth. Unlike measles there is no introductory phase and the rash is usually the first sign that your child has chicken pox. The typical rash may be preceded by a reddish diffuse rash. The disease is highly infective and the child is infective from the day the rash appears, for about a week. The crusts themselves are not infective. Having had chicken pox the child is very unlikely to have it again as a single infection usually confers immunity for life.

As in measles, the mouth can be involved and small blisters appear. These all rupture, leaving small shallow ulcers. But the main rash occurs on the body, usually developing on the back and chest first, although it may appear anywhere including the face and hands. The blisters do not usually appear on the soles of the feet or on the palms of the hands. The typical spot is an oval blister which eventually crusts over and then, when healed, leaves an oval white scar. The spots come in crops so that, although some of the spots may have crusted over, others may still be appearing. Although, commonly, many blisters appear, it is quite possible to have a very mild illness with very few blisters. And, in contrast to measles, the child himself generally does not feel too unwell and, indeed, may never develop a temperature.

The worst thing about the rash is that it may be intensely itchy and the child must be discouraged from scratching. It is wise to keep his fingernails really short so that he cannot scratch so effectively and simple calamine lotion may be helpful in stopping the worst of the itch, especially at night.

Severe complications of chicken pox are less common than with measles. But, occasionally, secondary infection such as impetigo can occur when scratching leaves open wounds. Very rarely, encephalitis can occur.

The virus of chicken pox is identical with that of shingles, or herpes zoster, to give it its official name. Children, therefore, who come into contact with an adult with shingles, may develop chicken pox. And, less commonly, adults who come into contact with children with chicken pox may develop shingles.

3 *Mumps*

This is another common infectious disease caused by a virus which affects the glands that produce saliva. It is caught by direct contact with infective droplets from the nose or mouth. It is very rare indeed in the first two years of life and is commonest between five and ten years. It is not as infective as measles or chicken pox, but a child who has it may infect others from two days before the swelling appears, until after it has completely disappeared.

Commonly, the first sign of mumps is the swelling itself, which is often on one side only, initially, although it usually spreads to the other side later. Occasionally, the child may be unwell, with a temperature, for a few days before the swelling appears. But, again, unlike measles, he does not feel unduly ill at any time during the illness. He will be off his food, partly because it becomes painful to bite, and partly because the infection decreases the supply of saliva leaving the mouth dry. The diagnosis depends upon the swelling itself which, characteristically, spreads up behind the ear pushing the ear lobe forward. The swelling may last several weeks and a second attack is very rare, a single attack usually conferring lifelong immunity.

The complications of mumps are well known, but very rarely affect a child. The virus can affect the testicles, but rarely before a boy reaches puberty. Secondary infection of the pancreas is rare in childhood. Mumps encephalitis, or meningitis, is seen as a complication of adult mumps but, there again, occurs very rarely in childhood.

As with all these virus infections, if the child feels unwell, he should be in bed. And the other single most important contribution to his happiness, is to keep his mouth moist with frequent drinks. As with any cause of illness in children, it is unwise to try to force solid food if the child obviously does not want it.

Because of the risk of boys becoming sterile if their testicles are involved if they get mumps after puberty, they should be encouraged to have the disease early on in childhood, if possible.

4   German Measles (rubella)

This is a mild infectious disease caused by a virus. It is commonest in the spring and is transmitted by direct contact with infected droplets. It may occur at any age and, because of the danger of women having the disease during pregnancy, girls should be actively encouraged to have it while they are young. The disease does not cause a lot of symptoms and, in fact, the child may hardly be ill at all. He might have a slight sore throat or runny nose and occasionally the eyes will weep, but nothing like as severely as in the case of measles. The rash consists of largish pale-pink spots, very widespread over the face, behind the ears, over the body and limbs and it fades fairly quickly leaving no discoloration or scarring. The characteristic sign of the disease is the appearance of enlarged glands predominantly up the back of the neck, although other glands can sometimes be felt.

Contrary to popular belief, German measles probably does not occur more than once. But the rash of the disease may be very easily confused with the rashes of other virus diseases, allergic drug rashes and milder cases of measles itself.

5 *Polio*

In spite of extensive immunisation, polio does still occur. It is a virus infection which is taken in by way of the mouth, after touching infected food or milk, or directly in crowded places such as swimming baths during an epidemic. Cases occur every year, but, whereas they used to be confined to the young child, they do now increasingly affect adults and adolescents. It occurs in three forms. There is the abortive form which is very rarely recognised, except in cases of acute epidemic, as it consists mainly of headaches, temperature and vomiting which are the symptoms of many other virus infections.

When these symptoms are accompanied by signs of meningitis with neck stiffness, it is called the 'non-paralytic' form.

The third form and the one that causes all the anxiety, is the 'paralytic' form. This is characterised by a first stage of being generally unwell with a sore throat, fever and aching limbs. There is then a latent period of about a week and the second or paralytic phase follows. This may be mild or severe. The course and management of the disease at this stage is very variable and will always require the child being in hospital. The important facts from the ordinary parents' point of view are: a) do have your child immunised, and b) do take all precautions should there be an epidemic in your area. It is very unwise, for example, to allow swimming in a public swimming bath if there is a local case of polio.

6 Scarlet Fever

This is an infection due to a specific streptococcus. It is commoner in older children than infants and is transmitted by direct droplet infection. It starts as an acute illness with a very high temperature, shivering, aches and pains, and with the throat feeling very dry. Then the characteristic throat appears, being red all over the mouth, but with thick white matter over the tonsils. A day or so after these symptoms, the rash appears as bright red spots over a generally reddened skin on the neck and chest. The rash can then spread all over the body and may last up to a week. As the rash heals, small areas of skin flake off, but these are not infective. The child is often described as being typically white around the mouth, while his body is red.

The tongue goes through three stages: a) the 'strawberry' tongue—the tongue is white and furred, but little red spots on it give it a truly strawberry-like appearance; b) the 'flaking' tongue —the white fur gradually flakes off; c) the 'raspberry' tongue— the tongue is bright red and smooth with raised bright red lumps on it.

These signs and symptoms are usually sufficient to make the diagnosis. But this cannot be made with absolute certainty unless the stretpococcus can be isolated from the throat. And, unfortunately from a diagnostic point of view, as the preceding symptoms are usually severe, penicillin will usually be given straightaway.

In young children, ear infections can be associated with scarlet fever. Because of the very high temperature, convulsions may occur in susceptible children. And, rarely, an allergic reaction to the streptococcus may occur which can cause acute rheumatic fever, or acute kidney disease. Because of these dangers, penicillin should be given in adequate dosage in any severe throat infection, even if a precise diagnosis cannot be made. At the same time, Aspirin may be given to make the child more comfortable and to reduce his temperature.

7 Whooping Cough

This is a common infectious disease caused by a small germ or bacillus which occurs mainly in very young children. It may occur in the first few months, as babies are not born with any immunity to it. It occurs most commonly in the spring and is spread by droplets from the infected person, either directly, or indirectly via toys or books which are then touched. A child may have a second or third attack.

The full course of the disease is very long and may be divided into three main parts. The first is an ordinary 'cold' stage with a runny nose, an annoying dry cough, occurring mainly at night, and, occasionally, a low fever. This can last up to two weeks. The typical 'whooping' phase can then last up to six weeks. The child gives a series of short coughs outwards while the breath is held and then, at the end, takes a long, characteristically 'whooping', breath inwards. These attacks may occur every hour or so and often end in vomiting and the unconscious passing of urine. The attacks are very exhausting and may be brought on by the slightest emotion or exercise.

The older child can cope with this most exhausting of diseases much more easily, but the real danger lies with the child under six months who gets the illness. Convulsions and pneumonia may occur as complications of the disease. The vaccinated child can get the disease, but if he does it is of a very much milder nature and the 'whoop' is not usually present.

The incidence of whooping cough has been declining for many years, probably mainly due to better living conditions. Vaccination against whooping cough has now been practised for many years and there is at present a great controversy over: (a) its effectiveness, and (b) whether it can be blamed for cases of severe brain damage that have occurred after it has been given. A full discussion on this may be found in the next section.

Apart from any discussion on vaccination, it is essential that young babies, particularly those under six months, should never be allowed to come into contact with any case of whooping cough. A young baby simply cannot cope with the exhaustion of the coughing and the thick mucus that has to be brought up with the cough.

8 *Roseola infantum*

I have included this here because it is a common infection of very young babies which can produce an alarming temperature, but which is of little danger to the child. Apart from the very high temperature which often reaches 105°F, there is little to show, apart, perhaps, from mild cold symptoms. The child does not appear unduly unwell. The fever lasts for four to five days and then, as it drops abruptly, a fine pink rash appears, covering most of the body, but not the face. It lasts two or three days and then fades, leaving no signs. There is no treatment and the child suffers no ill effects.

9 *Smallpox*

This disease is virtually non-existent in this country today. For this reason, no routine vaccination is now given, although it is still required for certain countries abroad. In view of the rarity of the disease I will not discuss it further here.

10 *Diphtheria*

Similarly, this disease, also due to widespread and effective immunisation, is virtually non-existent in this country.

Immunisation

Of all the subjects in this book none is of such topical importance as this. And this is simply because of the controversy at present surrounding the whooping cough vaccine. There is little variation in the rest of the infant immunisation from area to area and on the whole it seems to be effective and to cause little problem.

Diphtheria and tetanus are offered as a combined injection, starting the course sometime between three and six months. The second injection is given six to eight weeks after the first. And the third and final injection is given six months after the second. At the same time, polio immunisation is carried out. This comes as drops of liquid given direct in a tiny baby or on a sugar lump to an older child. Diphtheria, tetanus and polio are repeated as a pre-school booster at about four years.

Measles vaccination is offered at some time during the second year, preferably at least two months after the last combined diphtheria and tetanus.

Smallpox vaccination is no longer given routinely in this country as the side effects of the vaccination were found to be greater than the incidence of the disease would merit. Your doctor can still arrange for it to be done if you have to travel overseas to countries where it is mandatory.

These are the only immunisations carried out routinely within the age group discussed in this book. However, the BCG is offered at secondary school, and vaccination against rubella (German measles) is also offered to secondary-school girls between the ages of eleven and fourteen. For those women who have not been immunised, rubella vaccination is again offered immediately after delivery if the mother is found never to have had German measles.

It is interesting, and important, to know what substances are being given to your children especially in the light of present controversy. The protection against diphtheria is in the form of a toxoid which has been prepared from the toxin produced by the actual bacillus that causes diphtheria. The toxoid is joined on to a chemical substance which makes it safer and easier to use. Immunisation with the substance may cause the child to be slightly off colour for twenty-four to forty-eight hours. He may have a slight temperature. The site of the injection may go red and a small lump may form at the injection site feeling like a hard pea under the skin.

The protection against tetanus is, again, in the form of a toxoid and, in fact, diphtheria and tetanus are prepared together as a single injection for the primary immunisation of infants. Again, a transient rise in temperature may occur and the child may feel unwell for a day or two. Slight local redness and soreness is common. But it always resolves spontaneously and requires no treatment.

Very occasionally a child will be allergic to the vaccines, but this is very rare.

The protection against polio is a pale pink watery substance which contains attenuated forms of three strains of polio virus. It is readily taken by mouth mixed with something nice, such as a sugar solution or jam for younger children, whereas older children take it readily on a sugar lump. Side effects are very rare indeed.

Measles vaccine is a single injection of attenuated virus. It may produce symptoms like a mild attack of measles itself, between six and ten days after the injection. The child may be off-colour with a temperature, be very fretful and may even develop a few spots. Measles vaccine should not be given to a child with any history of convulsions in himself or his family.

BCG stands for Bacillus-Calmette-Guerin which are the names of the scientists who first isolated this particular strain of tubercle bacillus, occurring in cattle. The vaccine is the living bacilli which produce an active immunity to the bacillus of tuberculosis, within eight, or a maximum of fourteen, weeks. It should not be given within one month of any other vaccine containing living organisms.

Rubella or German measles vaccine is again a live attenuated virus and it may be given at any age. It should never be given to pregnant women or to any woman who could possibly become pregnant within two months of vaccination. Women who have never had rubella may be vaccinated against it immediately after the birth of their child to avoid risk during further pregnancies.

So I can now present a reasonable timetable of immunisation:

Age 3–6 months	diphtheria, tetanus, and oral polio
6–8 weeks later	diphtheria, tetanus, and oral polio
5–6 months later	diphtheria, tetanus, and oral polio
2–4 months later	measles injection
Age 4–4½ years	diphtheria, tetanus, and oral polio
Secondary school	BCG, rubella (girls only)

There remains the question of whooping cough vaccine. This has been given for a number of years as the third part of a combined injection with diphtheria and tetanus. The injection contains not more than 20,000 million chemically killed whooping cough organisms which are called bordatella pertussis. The controversy at present is over some cases of encephalitis, resulting in severe brain damage and mental retardation which seem to have a direct relationship with the injection. There seems no doubt that some of these cases, and they are rare, have been the direct result of whooping cough vaccination. The question remains as to whether the risk, small though it is, is justified in the prevention of whooping cough which can be a killer disease itself in the very young.

Statistics show that the incidence of whooping cough has been declining steadily and has continued to decline since the introduction of the immunisation programme. It is probable that the incidence of the disease would have continued to decline without the vaccine, but it is just possible that if we stop the vaccine the disease may reappear in epidemic proportions. There is no way that we can discover this without stopping the vaccine for a prescribed period of time.

There is no doubt that whooping cough vaccine should never

be given to any young child with a history of fits in himself or his family. It should never be given to a child who had cerebral irritation or 'twitching' episodes in the newborn period. It should never be given to children who are unwell at the time for any reason at all. It should never be given to those children with a history of allergy in themselves or in their families. And, again it should never be given to any child who has had any reaction whatsoever to a first dose.

The earlier time of starting the immunisation programme at three months was introduced because of the inclusion of the whooping cough vaccine. The earlier a child gets whooping cough the greater is the danger of the disease. However, there is evidence that immunity to these diseases is built up more efficiently if the immunisation programme is deferred until nearer 6 months.

In the light of the present facts and controversy, I can see no alternative, but to stop routine whooping cough vaccination and to measure the increase or decline of the disease. If the disease does show a marked increase in incidence, then obviously whooping cough vaccine should be re-introduced with a, hopefully, improved vaccine and with the strict provisos in the paragraph above.

Your Social Baby—His Activities and Play

There is no doubt that even a very young baby loves company. Very early on he will love another baby playing on the floor with him. But he will have no idea of sharing toys at all. However, I am sure that wide social contacts from a very early age do help him to adjust more quickly to an active enjoyment of play with other children later on. But you cannot force the pace and expect him to cope if he is left alone with other unfamiliar people too early. Within the age range of the scope of this book, toddler playgroups should be with mothers, unless your child shows a remarkable independence early on.

There are more toys on the market now than any of us will ever be in a position to afford. So do choose new toys wisely. It is always quoted that children get more enjoyment out of, for instance, an old shopping basket filled with oddments, such as pegs, cotton reels, empty cartons etc, than out of any expensive toys. This is certainly true to some extent. But the wise buying of some toys can enlarge his field of play and his interest greatly. The first things that you will buy are the rattles. Do make sure that these have handles that are small enough for very small hands to grasp. Do make sure that the colours are clear and bright but not phosphorescent. And, finally, do make sure that the rattle itself is musical. You must remember that the baby will be rattling the toy very close to his ear and nothing is worse than a noise that is not only ugly but too loud. Children love putting things in and out of other things. So when your baby is ready to progress from the rattle stage, invest in the cups or barrels of graded sizes. These are usually brightly coloured and very attractive. They can be used as receptacles, for building castles and for all sorts of other games. Toys where rings are threaded onto a central handle, or toys of the post-box variety, where different shapes must be matched to different holes, develop hands and mind, and the co-ordination of both well. One large ball can provide much enjoyment. As soon as your child is pulling to his feet, do afford a trolley of bricks. The bricks will last as playthings for years in different forms of play and the trolley will be a great stimulus for walking. Do save all your empty plastic bottles and yoghurt cups for bath play and sand and dirt play. Books that you get early on should be large, thick-paged and have brightly coloured pictures of readily identified objects.

Finally, do not be tempted to buy beautiful, complicated and expensive toys such as dolls' houses and garages too early. You will only be disappointed as your child fails to play with them in the adult way that you think the toys deserve. So wait until he is ready for those. Early on, have a few large, durable, washable and safe toys and let him invent his own play during the first few years. There are always many Christmases and birthdays to come for buying more toys.

Prevention of Accidents

Accidents still form a very high proportion of the deaths in childhood. It is worthwhile reminding ourselves continually of the commoner causes.

1 *Drugs and Medicines*

1 Never leave any pills, drugs, or medicines within reach at any time, even for a few minutes. Medicines should be in a locked cupboard high up out of reach; and remember that children learn to climb upon chairs very quickly. A few moments is enough for the damage to be done. I have seen an Aspirin bottle emptied while a mother answered the phone.

2 If you discover that your toddler has eaten tablets or medicine, tell your doctor immediately, or, if he is unavailable, go to the casualty department of your nearest hospital straightaway.

3 If you know the child has taken Aspirin then, if you can get him to vomit, it is well worth it. But if you do not know what it is, do not waste time in trying to make a child vomit; get him to hospital immediately.

2 *Household Fluids and Garden Poisons*

Again the rule is simple, but it is all too easy to make mistakes.

1 Never leave an active and inquisitive child alone.

2 Keep all household things out of reach.

3 Go to the hospital immediately if you are at all unsure.

4 Never try to make him vomit if there is any possibility that acids, alkalis, or paraffin have been taken.

5 Wash off any acids or chemicals that have been spilt with water and leave the skin, if affected, uncovered.

3 Burns and Scalds

The rules again must be obvious:

1   Never leave a child alone in the kitchen.

2   Never leave a fire unguarded. The guard should be substantial and should completely surround the fire. Never leave him alone in a room with an open fire. Put him in a play-pen or take him with you when you answer the phone or the door.

3   Never leave matches accessible.

4   Never boil a kettle on the floor. Remember that steam burns are worse than those caused by boiling water.

If your child should get burnt or scalded:

1   Minor scalds should be washed off with water and then Acriflex, or a similar cream, should be applied.

2   With any burn or scald, that is worse than very slight, all clothing should be removed from the affected part.

3   Any burning fluid or fat should be washed off with water immediately.

4   Do not try to cover it.

5   Seek medical help from your doctor or the nearest hospital immediately.

4 Stairs

Of course, at some time your baby must learn to go up and down stairs. If you are lucky you will have the sort of staircase that has two or three steps separated from the main flight. This means that you will be able to barricade off the main flight and teach your baby on the comparative safety of just two or three steps. But, whatever your staircase arrangements, you must prevent your child taking that tumble from top to bottom. And this usually means providing a gate across the stairs at the bottom when you are downstairs and, perhaps more important, at the top when you are upstairs.

5 Falling

1   Never leave a baby unguarded in a high chair. If you have

to be in and out of a room, then you must strap him in.

2   Never leave him unattended on a table, bed, or chair. It only requires you to turn your back for one second for him to fall off.

3   Remember that things can fall off on to him as well as he himself falling off. Do keep tablecloths out of reach. One quick pull will bring the entire contents of the table onto his head, including hot teapots.

6   Knives and Scissors

These should never be left within reach, not so much because of the damage that they can do in the hand, but because if they are carried around and the child falls on them, they can do untold damage. Never let a child walk or run with anything sharp in his hand or, worse, his mouth.

7   Toys

Do make sure that the toys you buy, or those that you are given, are safe:

1   The paint on toys must be free of lead. Lead poisoning does still occur.

2   Do make sure that there are no sharp ends or metal pieces on the toy.

3   Fluffy toys and dolls have eyes and buttons. Particularly with a young baby, do make sure these are not removable.

4   Do not give small bricks, marbles or other toys to young children who still tend to put things in their mouths.

5   Do not leave toys in cots. Do not provide pillows in cots for young babies.

8   Windows

Upstairs bedroom windows particularly must be provided with bars, and all catches must be foolproof. A baby cannot be relied upon not to climb on window sills and to fiddle with the catches. And do remember that, even if your children are completely trustworthy, if they have young friends staying with them, they may do things they would not dream of doing when they are alone.

9 Roads

If you do leave your children playing in the garden, do make sure that they cannot stray on to the road. Do not let them play on or near roads. And when you are out walking in a town, make sure that young children are on reins or in a pushchair.

10 Playgrounds

For some extraordinary reason playgrounds are almost uniformly constructed of concrete. Do not let a child who is not old, or sensible, enough follow his older brothers and sisters onto climbing frames. And do watch out for, perhaps, the greatest hazard of playgrounds, the swings. Time and again children receive bad head injuries from being hit by another child swinging because they will run right in front of the swing.

11 Cars and Car Seats

There is absolutely no doubt that children are safer travelling in the back seat and that the younger child should be strapped into a safety-approved car seat. It can be difficult to amuse the older child on a long journey but he should be taught to sit and not stand up. And there is no doubt that if you are driving with children and no other adults, you should have your children in car seats where at all possible.

12 Plants and Berries

There are more berries in the hedgerow that are dangerous than not. So the only safe rule is not to allow any berries to be put anywhere near a child's mouth.

13 Bathrooms

Do not leave your child alone in the bath or, indeed, by a pond or stream. The water does not need to be deep to drown a small child.

14 *Holidays and the Sea*

Every year there continue to be accidents, several fatal, on holiday and particularly on the beaches.

1   Do not expose a young child to excessive sun the first day of your seaside holiday.

2   Do use a good child-approved sun cream, particularly for a child with a fair skin. And use it *before* the child gets sunburnt. Fair-skinned children should wear a hat on the beach. If your child's skin does begin to burn, cover him with a light T-shirt. You do not need to leave the beach.

3   Do not lose sight of your children on the beach. It is all too easy to get lost and for a child to wander far away.

4   Do make sure of local tides and currents. Do listen to the advice of local lifeguards. They are not trying to spoil your holiday. They know what they are talking about.

5   Never let your children go into the sea alone (unless of course they are older and good swimmers).

6   Do not use inflatable mattresses and dinghies unless you are personally in charge and, preferably, have them on a life-line.

7   Never let your children take out a dinghy alone.

8   Do not let your children run about wildly at the edge of a cliff.

9   Always take note of local warning signs.

10   It is always wise to carry with you a small number of Elastoplast dressings, sunburn cream, and Anthisan cream, or something similar, for the treatment of bites and stings.

INDEX

JAN HOPCRAFT

Cooking Today, Eating Tomorrow

Do you like to cook for your friends but always find yourself too rushed to enjoy it? This bestselling cookery book is designed for busy people. The recipes are clearly presented in the form of menus for dinner, lunch and fork supper parties. No menu contains more than one dish which has to be made from start to finish on the actual day. Each recipe has been specially designed to cut right down on time spent in the kitchen at the last minute, so that you can enjoy more time with your guests.

'A useful book for anyone who enjoys entertaining but dreads the last-minute flap in the kitchen'
House and Garden

Entertaining on a Budget

A practical guide to tempting yet inexpensive meals for entertaining. Jan Hopcraft demonstrates that lashings of wine and cream are not essential for a first-class meal. She uses cider and a wide range of herbs and spices to transform simple ingredients into delicious and exciting dishes. These imaginative recipes include totally new ideas as well as traditional dishes and advice on cutting costs. Many dishes can be prepared in advance, making this an essential cookery book for those who have to economise on time as well as cost.

CAROLYN McCRUM

The Soup Book

Soup is a versatile food suitable for all occasions. A delicate consommé will make a fine start to a rich meal; an iced soup is wonderfully refreshing on a summer's day; and a meat soup can satisfy the heartiest appetite as a complete meal on a winter's night.

In *The Soup Book* Carolyn McCrum explains the basic methods and essential equipment for stock and soup-making. There are many recipes ranging from simple soups that can be prepared in minutes, to elaborate soups like the famed Bouillabaise, Pot-au-Feu and Gazpacho. Favourite soups are included as well as new ideas, such as Iced Coconut and Aubergine Soup. The recipes are arranged practically for particular occasions: time-saving soups, cool summer soups, and main course soups for family suppers.

The Soup Book will persuade you that the soup you make yourself is infinitely superior to the processed kind: it is delicious, nourishing, wonderfully versatile and a pleasure to prepare.

ROSEMARY STARK

The Miracle Cookbook

Most of us experience at some time or other that sinking feeling when guests turn up unexpectedly for a meal. Panic no more, for Rosemary Stark comes to the rescue with a wealth of ideas for improvisation in the kitchen, By adding an extra course or expanding what's to hand with goodies from the store cupboard, you can even stretch two pork chops between four people.

JEAN CONIL

The Magnum Cookbook

The Magnum Cookbook is a must for all serious cooks. It contains a wide variety of recipes ranging from the basic to the exotic, as well as exciting recipes for special occasions. Roast beef and Yorkshire pudding and a host of other traditional English recipes are included.

Master Chef Jean Conil's experience as a chef and nutritionist has enabled him to write a comprehensive book covering all aspects of cookery. He outlines the basic 'do's' and 'don'ts' of which every cook should be aware; a knowledge which he hopes will give confidence and inspiration to develop new ideas in the kitchen.

Jean Conil has had a varied career as a chef, restaurateur, author and teacher.

ROGER GROUNDS
The Natural Garden

The Natural Garden argues that everything in your garden is natural; worm populations and mulches will produce good soil, and in the long run the natural predators of insects will control their spread. This way, your garden will be healthier, fruits and vegetables will look and taste better, and plants will flower more beautifully.

ROGER GROUNDS & ROBIN HOWE
Fresh from the Garden

Just think how much more delicious your food could be if you use vegetables and fruit fresh from your own garden! Roger Grounds and Robin Howe have collaborated to provide a complete book for everyone who wants to grow and cook their own vegetables and fruit.

Roger Grounds, an enthusiastic natural gardener, gives advice on the best possible way to grow your vegetables and fruit. His main concern is to achieve the best flavour. Robin Howe, an experienced cookery writer, has lived in various parts of the world. Here, she offers many exciting and imaginative recipes which will bring out the full flavour of your home-grown produce. An additional chapter by Brenda Sanctuary provides a complete guide to freezing, so that you can enjoy your own vegetables through the year.

GILLIAN PEARKS

Complete Home Wine-making

If you think home wine-making is a complicated and messy process with an inferior end-product, then this book will show you that it is not. It is a fascinating and relatively simple pursuit, inexpensive to engage in with richly rewarding results. For those who already enjoy the art of home wine-making there are many new and exciting recipes for all kinds of wine: fresh-fruit wine, dried-fruit wine, flower wine, cereal wine, vegetable wine, and also cider, mead, perry and liqueurs.

From your first cautious step into home wine-making this book guides you through to the most ambitious wines.

BOB SENNETT

The International Drinker's Companion

Here is the complete and definitive handbook on the fine art of creating the perfect cocktail. Encyclopaedic in scope, the Companion has a place in every party-giver's home and is an essential reference tool for the professional bartender. Even if you've never mixed a drink in your life, you'll find that the easy instructions will enable you to produce a perfect result the very first time. Each drink recipe is illustrated with the appropriate glass, and the book contains special sections on: the home bar, the professional cocktail bar, tips for bartenders, bar equipment and glasses and liqueurs.

GEOFFREY NICHOLSON
The Great Bike Race

The Tour de France is the greatest annual sports event in the world. A gruelling 25-day, 2,500-mile journey, it encircles the country, cuts across frontiers and climbs the Alps to 8,000 feet. Geoffrey Nicholson has written a personal journal focused on a single Tour. He describes the personalities, tactics, intrigues and the bizarre commercial background to the 1976 race. He writes about the legends which have built up around the Tour and tries to discover why the French are so obsessed by this annual bike race.

ANTHONY BURTON
Back Door Britain

Back Door Britain is the fascinating story of a thousand-mile journey of discovery, a canal and river voyage which took the author into the secret centres of towns and cities and through the beauties of the open countryside. Humorous and yet packed with practical information, it offers the reader a remarkable inside view of the delights and surprises of back door Britain.

'The reader cannot help but be affected by his enthusiasm'

Motor Boat and Yachting

'Outward-going, loudly delighting in discovery and experience; opinionated in a healthy way; and with a talent for giving us the flavour of places'

The Times